Surgical Case-Histories from the Past

Harold Ellis
CBE FRCS

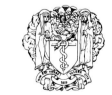

Royal Society of Medicine Press

Royal Society of Medicine Press Limited
1 Wimpole Street   London W1M 8AE
150 East 58th Street   New York NY 10155

British Library Cataloguing in Publication Data
A catalogue record for this book is available from the British Library

ISBN 1-85315-222-6

Photypeset by Dobbie Typesetting Limited, Tavistock, Devon
Printed in Great Britain by Ebenezer Baylis, The Trinity Press, Worcester

Contents

III Surgical Emergencies and Disasters

IV The Surgeon At Work

Acknowledgements

A good number of these 'Surgical Case-Histories from the Past' have appeared, in more abbreviated form, over the past few years, in *Contemporary Surgery* in the USA and in *Surgery* in the UK. I would like to thank Dr Seymour Schwartz and Mrs Peggy Plendl of the former, and Mr John Craven, FRCS and Mrs Jill McFarland of the latter Journal for their encouragement to publish this collection in book form.

Mr Ian Lyle, Tina Craig and the rest of the staff at the library of the Royal College of Surgeons of England and Mrs Barbie Wells of the library of the Department of Anatomy of the University of Cambridge were of immense help in my search for original texts and illustrations. I wish to thank the photographic units of the Anatomy Departments in Cambridge and the United Medical and Dental Schools at Guy's and the secretaries in these two Departments, Miss Sarah Clark and Mrs Sheila Bishop respectively, for their skilled and cheerful help.

Assistance with individual case reports came from many sources. I particularly wish to thank for the following:

Case (6) Jonathan Hutchinson—Mr Jonathan Evans (Archivist at the Royal London Hospital)

(9) Carl Langenbuch—Professor KJ Hardy (Melbourne)

(11) Henry Souttar—Professor John Blandy

(12) Charles Dubost—Mrs Jennifer York (Paris)

(15) Thomas Eshelby—Surgeon Captain IL Evans RN and Professor John Trounce

(22) Astley Cooper—Professor Norman Browse, PRCS

(25) Augustus Eves—Miss Daphne Daughton, SRN and Mrs Maryse Roberts (Cheltenham Postgraduate Centre)

(29) Lorenz Heister—Dr William Beck (Sayr, USA)

(30) John Hunter—Miss Elizabeth Allen (Curator, Hunterian Museum, Royal College of Surgeons of England)

(35) Jaques Louis Reverdin—Dr Guy Saudan (Pully, Switzerland).

I acknowledge permission to reproduce case reports from the following Journals:

Archives of Surgery, and *La semaine des Hôpitaux* (Charles Dubost, Case 12)
The Lancet (Grey Turner, Case 17, and anonymous Case 20)
British Medical Journal (Henry Souttar, Case 11).

The sources of the illustrations are acknowledged in their subtitles.

Finally, I wish to thank Mr Howard Croft and his staff at the Royal Society of Medicine Publications for their patient help in the preparation of this Volume.

For our grandsons—
Jordan and Jack

Introduction

As long as there have been medical records, so there have been case reports of patients. Indeed, there has always seemed to be the desire of doctors to document their interesting cases. The teaching of medicine down the ages has also relied heavily on anecdotes of particular patients. Moreover the tyro surgeon or physician builds up his clinical experience from his personal contact with individual sufferers.

The earliest known surgical treatise, the Edwin Smith Papyrus, in fact, consists of no less than the details of 48 cases of wounds and fractures. It dates from about the year 1550 BC but it was undoubtedly a copy of a more ancient text. These cases commence at the head and work downwards; a classification commonly employed in Greek and later medical books. The text is incomplete and breaks off in mid sentence at the thorax. The original book, of which the Edwin Smith Papyrus is a partial copy, might well have been complete.

Each case is presented as a title, examination, diagnosis, verdict ('an ailment to treat, an ailment to contend, or an ailment not to be treated') and treatment.

As an example of these earliest known case reports, case 40 is as follows:

'Instructions concerning a wound in his breast.

If thou examinest a man having a wound in his breast, penetrating to the bone, perforating the manubrium of his sternum, thou shouldst press the manubrium of his sternum with thy fingers, although he shudders exceedingly.

Though shouldst say concerning him: "One having a wound in his breast penetrating to the bone, perforating the manubrium of his sternum. An ailment which I will treat."

Thou shouldst bind it with fresh lint the first day: thou shouldst treat it afterward with grease, honey and lint every day until he recovers.'

The Hippocratic writings of the fifth century B.C. contain numerous case reports, especially in the book of Epidemics. For example, case 9 reads: 'The woman who lodged at the house of Tisamenas had a troublesome attack of iliac passion, much vomiting; could not keep her drink; pains about the hypochondria and pains also in the lower part of the belly; constant tormina; not thirst; became hot; extremities cold throughout, with nausea and insomnolency; urine scanty and thin; dejections undigested, thin, scanty. Nothing could do her any good. She died.'

This sounds like a good description of peritonitis in this translation by Francis Adams, perhaps as a result of a perforated appendix.

The vivid descriptions that have come down to us in books and articles from our surgical forefathers give a wonderful picture of the art and craft of surgery through the centuries. However, to appreciate these reports, it is important for the reader to transfer himself to the degree of knowledge at the time of the case report. It is easy enough for us today to laugh at the term 'laudable pus' and wonder how surgeons could ever consider the discharge of purulent material from a wound to be a good thing. However, it is important to remember that before the microscope and the days of

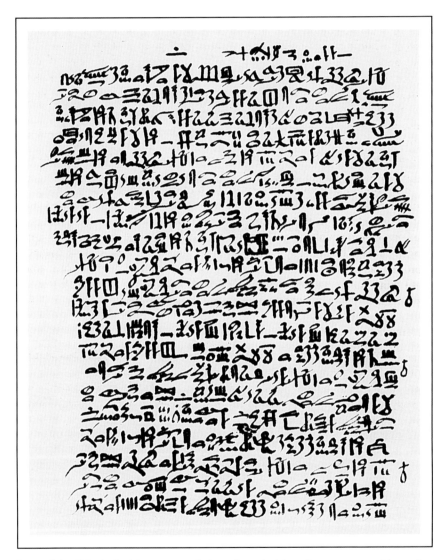

Part of the Edwin Smith papyrus. It is written in hieratic, a more rapid cursive form of hieroglyphic signs. The earliest known surgical case reports.
(From J. H. Breasted *Edwin Smith Surgical Papyrus* Chicago, University of Chicago Press 1930 with permission of the publishers)

Pasteur there was complete ignorance of the bacterial nature of wound infection. The surgeons of those days were shrewd observers. Following an open wound or a compound fracture, patients would often become seriously ill with fever, a rapid pulse, toxaemia and soon die. These, we now know, were the victims of overwhelming septicaemia. If pus appeared in the wound, we also now know, this was a manifestation of the body's local defences against bacterial invasion. His recovery might indeed be tedious but, at least, he had a chance of survival.

In this book, the case reports have been grouped into four sections. The first, and obvious, group comprises what are now so often referred to as 'major break-throughs'—the first report of an operation under general anaesthesia, the first cardiac massage or the first resection of an aortic aneurysm. The second group comprises descriptions by surgeons in battle, often struggling with scanty facilities under poor conditions to deal with large numbers of casualties. The third group is a collection of emergencies and disasters and the final section is made up of a miscellany of interesting patients, pathologies and operations.

Since surgery burgeoned in the second half of the 19th century, under the twin blessings of anaesthesia and antisepsis, and since living authors have not been included in this selection, it is not surprising that the majority of the reports in this volume are dated from the 1870s to the early 1900s. Some surgeon in the future may well produce a similar volume of case histories from the second half of the now dying 20th century and will collect a rich yield from the amazing advances that have been made in transplantation, replacement, reconstructive and minimal access surgery.

References

Adams F. *The Genuine Works of Hippocrates translated from the Greek.* Introduction by E. C. Kelly. Baltimore: Williams and Wilkins, 1939.
Breasted JH. *The Edwin Smith Surgical Papyrus. Published in facsimile and hieroglyphic transliteration with translation and commentary in two volumes.* Chicago: University of Chicago Press, 1930.

Part I
Major Advances

[1]

Ephraim McDowell

The first successful ovariotomy (1809)

It is an interesting exercise to ask a new entry of medical students if they can guess the date of the first successful elective laparotomy, the name of the surgeon who performed the operation and where it took place. After a long and profound silence, someone may tentatively suggest 'Around 1870 or 1880', guess at some well known name, such as Joseph Lister, (who, in fact, never opened the abdomen in his life), and opine that the venue must

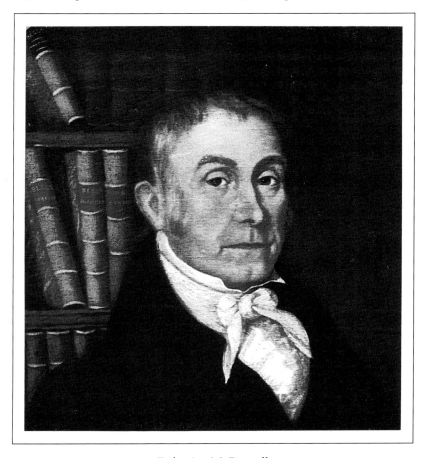

Ephraim McDowell
(Courtesy of the President, Royal College of Obstetricians and Gynaecologists, London)

have been a London teaching hospital or one of the great European Surgical Clinics. None of these could be further from the truth. The fact is the date was 1809, the surgeon Ephraim McDowell and the place Danville, Kentucky.

Ephraim McDowell was born in 1771 in Rockbridge County, Virginia, the great grandson of a Northern Irish Protestant who emigrated to the United States. His grandfather was killed in an Indian ambush and his father was a colonel in the Revolutionary War.

The family moved to Kentucky when Ephraim was 13 years of age, when his father was appointed a judge at Danville, the first capital of that state which, at that time, had 'upwards of 150 homes and some tolerably good buildings'. At the age of 19 he was apprenticed to Dr Alexander Humphreys at Staunton, Virginia and then spent two years in Edinburgh, where he attended the sessions of 1793 and 1794, following the anatomy lectures of Alexander Munro (secundus) and studying surgery under John Bell. By 1795 he was back in Danville as its only surgeon. He soon built up an extensive practice which covered hundreds of miles of frontier territory. Here a call could mean a long ride on horse-back in country where both Indians and wolves were still a threat. Rapidly he became the leading surgeon west of the Alleghenies.

Among McDowell's successes was that he carried out two lithotomies without a death; one of these was James K. Polk, who later became President of the United States of America.

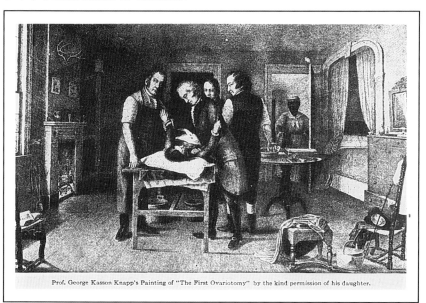

Prof. George Kasson Knapp's Painting of "The First Ovariotomy" by the kind permission of his daughter.

'The first ovariotomy'. Painting by Professor George Kasson Knappe. McDowell stands at the left of the painting
(From H. Ellis *Famous Operations* Media, Harwal 1983)

McDowell had a preference for operating on Sundays. Possibly this was because he liked to have the benefit of the prayers of the Church or possibly because it was the one quiet day of the week.

On December 13th 1809, McDowell was called to see Mrs Jane Todd Crawford, who lived with her family in a log cabin at Motley's Glen, Green County, then about 46 years of age and the mother of five children. As her case report describes, Mrs Crawford thought herself pregnant and to be in the last stage of pregnancy. Indeed, two physicians who were consulted on her case requested McDowell's aid in delivering her. After a pelvic examination, McDowell diagnosed a massive ovarian cyst and offered to carry out an experiment if she were able to reach Danville. Mrs Crawford undertook the journey on horse-back and laparotomy was duly performed in McDowell's front parlour without, of course, the benefit of any form of anaesthesia. McDowell was assisted by his nephew, Dr James McDowell, who had graduated a few months before in Philadelphia and who had joined the practice as a partner.

Within five days Mrs Crawford was up and about making her own bed and in 25 days she returned home in good health, again on horse-back, the 60 mile journey to her log cabin. She lived to the ripe old age of 78, dying in 1842 and having outlived her surgeon by 12 years.

McDowell did not publish his triumphant result immediately—the first elective laparotomy carried out successfully for an accurately diagnosed intra-abdominal pathology. Perhaps he was too diffident, or perhaps he did not realise the implications of the case. It may be that his busy practice gave him little time for writing and he was certainly not a particularly literary man. Whatever the reason, McDowell waited until he had performed two further successful ovariotomies, both on black women, before publishing his report in 1817. Two years later, he reported two further cases, again both black women. One was successful but the second patient died of peritonitis on the third post-operative day. Although McDowell published no more, he did continue to perform this operation. Between 1822 and 1826 he operated on three more women, all of them white. In one, the ovarian mass was incised and drained; the patient lived for a considerable time following this. The second involved complete excision and the third had to be abandoned because of extensive adhesions. There is evidence that McDowell performed at least 12 operations for ovarian pathology, but no details exist of the later cases.

It took some time for McDowell's successes to be accepted. He sent a copy of his first report to his old teacher, John Bell, in Edinburgh. Bell was then in Rome, where he died shortly after, so it was John Lizars, who became Professor of Surgery at the College of Surgeons of Edinburgh, who received the report. Lizars did nothing about the paper until his own publication *Observations on extraction of Diseased Ovaria* in 1825, in which he reported four cases, one of which was successful. In this report he quoted McDowell's paper, although by now two other American surgeons had performed successful ovariectomies—Nathan Smith in Connecticut in 1821 and A. G. Smith in Kentucky in 1823.

McDowell's first report was received with some scepticism. Thus, in an article in the London Medical and Chirurgical Review, Dr James Johnson wrote 'three cases of ovarian extirpation occurred, it would seem, some years ago in the practice of Dr McDowell of Kentucky, which were transmitted to the late John Bell and fell into the hands of Mr Lizars. We candidly confess we are rather sceptical respecting these statements, and we are rather surprised that Lizars himself should put implicit confidence in them'.

However, the publication of McDowell's second report made even the unbelieving English repent and, in 1826, the same author wrote: 'A back settlement of America—Kentucky—has beaten the mother country, nay Europe itself, with all the boasted surgeons thereof, in the fearful and formidable operation of gastrotomy, with extraction of diseased ovaria . . . there were circumstances in the narrative of some of the three cases that raised misgivings in our minds, for which uncharitableness we ask pardon of God and of Dr McDowell of Danville'.

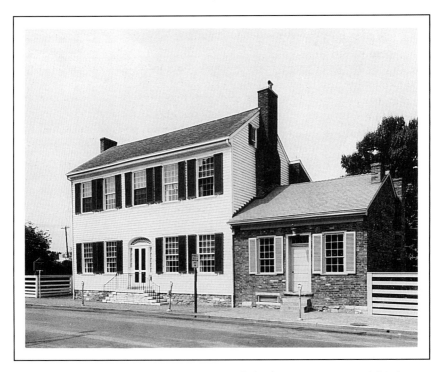

The house in which McDowell performed the first ovariotomy. This house is carefully preserved and is now a museum
(Courtesy of the President, Royal College of Obstetricians and Gynaecologists, London)

Since that time the stature of McDowell has grown in surgical history and he is now acknowledged as not only the father of ovariotomy but also of abdominal surgery.

McDowell died in 1830 at the age of 59 after a two week illness of 'an acute attack of inflammation of the stomach', perhaps acute appendicitis. What a pity that abdominal surgery had not progressed a little further at that time! McDowell was buried in the family burial ground. In 1879 his remains were removed to what is now called McDowell Park. The spot is marked by a fine memorial shaft on which the inscription reads 'Beneath this shaft rests Ephraim McDowell MD the father of ovariotomy, who by originating a great surgical operation became a benefactor of his race, known and honoured throughout the civilised world'.

Ephraim McDowell "Three cases of extirpation of diseased ovaria"

The Eclectic Repertory and Analytical Review 1817; 7: 242

'In December 1809, I was called to see a Mrs Crawford who had for several months thought herself pregnant. She was affected with pains similar to labour pains, from which she could find no relief. So strong was the presumption of her being in the last stage of pregnancy, that two physicians, who were consulted on her case, requested my aid in delivering her. The abdomen was considerably enlarged, and had the appearance of pregnancy, though the inclination of the tumour was to one side, admitting of an easy removal to the other. Upon examination, per vaginam, I found nothing in the uterus; which induced the conclusion that it must be an enlarged ovarium. Having never seen so large a substance extracted, nor heard of an attempt, or success attending any operation, such as this required, I gave to the unhappy woman information of her dangerous situation. She appeared willing to undergo an experiment, which I promised to perform if she would come to Danville (the town where I live), a distance of sixty miles from her place of residence. This appeared almost impracticable by any, even the most favourable conveyance, though she performed the journey in a few days on horseback. With the assistance of my nephew and colleague, James McDowell MD, I commenced the operation, which was concluded as follows: Having placed her on a table of the ordinary height, on her back, and removed all her dressing which might in any way impede the operation, I made an incision about three inches from the muscular rectus abdominis, on the left side, continuing the same nine inches in length, parallel with the fibres of the above named muscle, extending into the cavity of the abdomen, the parietes of which were a good deal contused, which we ascribed to the resting of the tumor on the horn of the saddle during her journey. The tumor then appeared full in view, but was so large that we could not take it away entire. We put a strong ligature around the fallopian tube near to the uterus; we then cut open the tumor, which was the ovarium and fimbrious part of the fallopian tube very much enlarged. We took out fifteen pounds of a dirty, gelatinous looking substance. After which we cut through the fallopian tube, and extracted the sack, which weighed seven pounds and one half. As soon as the external opening was made, the intestines rushed out upon the table; and so completely was the abdomen filled by the tumor, that they could not be replaced during the operation which was terminated in about twenty-five minutes. We then turned her upon her left side, so as to permit the blood to escape; after which we closed the external opening with the interrupted suture, leaving out at the lower end of the incision, the ligature which surrounded the fallopian tube. Between every two stitches we put a strip of adhesive plaster, which, by keeping the parts in contact, hastened the healing of the incision. We then applied the usual dressings, put her to bed, and prescribed a strict observance of the antiphlogistic regimen. In five days I visited her, and much to my astonishment found her engaged in making up her bed. I gave her particular caution for the future; and in twenty-five days, she returned home as she came, in good health which she continues to enjoy.

Since the case, I was called to a Negro woman, who had a hard and very painful tumor in the abdomen. I gave her mercury for three or four months with some abatement of pain; but she was still unable to perform her usual duties. As the tumor was fixed and immovable, I did not advise an operation; though from the earnest solicitation of her master, and her own distressful condition, I agreed to the experiment. I had her placed upon a table, laid her side open as in the above case; put my hand in, found the ovarium very much enlarged, painful to the touch, and firmly adhering to the vesica urinaria and fundus uteri. To extract I thought would be instantly fatal; but by way of experiment I plunged my scalpel into the diseased part. Such gelatinous substance as in the above case, with a profusion of blood, rushed to the external opening, and I conveyed it off by placing my hand under the tumor, and suffering the discharge to take place over it. Notwithstanding my great care, a quart or more of blood escaped into the abdomen. After the hemorrhage ceased, I took out as nearly as possible the blood, in which the bowels were completely enveloped. Though I considered the case as nearly hopeless, I advised the same dressings, and the same regimen as in the above case. She has entirely recovered from all pain, and pursues her ordinary occupations.

In May 1816, a Negro woman was brought to me from a distance. I found the ovarium much enlarged, and as it could easily be moved from side to side, I advised the extraction of it. As it adhered to the left side, I changed my place of opening to the linea alba. I began the incision, in company with my partner and colleague Dr William Coffer, an inch below the umbilicus, and extended it to within an inch of the os pubis. I then put a ligature around the fallopian tube and endeavoured to turn out the tumor, but could not. I then cut to the right of the umbilicus, and above it two inches, turned out a scirrhous ovarium (weighing six pounds), and cut it off close to the ligature, put round the fallopian tube. I then closed the external opening, as in the former cases; and she complaining of cold and chilliness, I put her to bed prior to dressing her—then gave her a wine glass full of cherry bounce, and thirty drops of laudanum, which soon restoring her warmth, she was dressed as usual. She was well in two weeks, though the ligature could not be released for five weeks; at the end of which time the cord was taken away; and she now, without complaint, officiates in the laborious occupation of cook to a large family.'

References

Ellis H. *Famous Operations*. Media, Harwal Publishing Co, 1984.

McDowell E. Three cases of extirpation of diseased ovaries. *The Eclectic Repertory and Analytical Review* 1817; 7: 242

Schachner A. *Ephraim McDowell: Father of Ovariotomy and Founder of Abdominal Surgery*. Philadelphia; Lippincott, 1921

Scott Earle A. *Surgery in America. From the Colonial Era to the Twentieth Century* 2nd edition. New York: Praeger, 1983

[2]

John Collins Warren

Operations under ether anaesthesia (1846)

The Professor of Surgery at Harvard in 1846, eminent though he was at the time, would be unknown to most of us today had he not performed a fairly trivial operation, the removal of a lump from the neck of a young lad called Gilbert Abbot. This minor procedure was, in fact, to be one of the most important landmarks in surgical history, because it was the first time that an operation was performed in public under the influence of ether.

The date, October 16th, 1846, was the watershed between the past agonies of the surgical knife, mitigated only by alcohol or opium, and the modern era, when the patients enjoy the blissful oblivion of anaesthesia.

The place, the old theatre of the Massachusetts General Hospital in Boston, below the central dome of the old building, is carefully preserved today and named 'The Ether Dome'.

John Collins Warren (1778–1856) was the son of Dr John Warren, the first Professor of Surgery at Harvard. He was born in Boston, studied medicine with his father, learned his surgery under Astley Cooper at Guy's Hospital

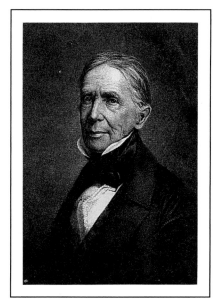
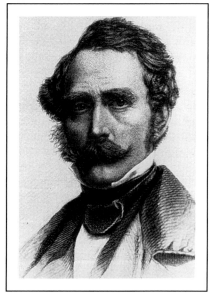

John Collins Warren   William Morton

(From B. MacQuitty *Battle for Oblivion* London, Harrap 1969)

London, took the Edinburgh M.D. in 1801, studied in Paris under the great Baron Dupuytren, practised with his father and then succeeded him as second Professor of Surgery at Harvard in 1815. Among his important accomplishments was that he helped to found the Massachusetts General Hospital and the New England Journal of Medicine and Surgery (as it was first called, it was only later that 'Surgery' was dropped from the title). Warren also wrote the first American text book on tumours.

The real hero of the day, William Thomas Green Morton (1819–1868), was a Boston dentist, then aged 27, who had experimented with the use of ether in the successful mitigation of the pain of dental extractions. Morton approached Warren to allow him the opportunity of exhibiting his drug to surgical patients, and it is to Warren's eternal credit that, as a very senior man of 68, he allowed this young fellow the opportunity of a public demonstration. The authority of Warren made the immediate acceptance of ether a certainty.

Morton's apparatus had progressed from a handkerchief soaked in ether, in his first dental extractions, to a two-necked glass globe. One neck allowed the inflow of air, the other, fitted with a wooden mouth piece, permitted the subject to inhale air across the surface of an ether-soaked sponge inside the globe.

All the anxieties of an important clinical trial are summed up by Morton's young wife, who later wrote:

'The night before the operation my husband worked until 1 or 2 o'clock in the morning upon the inhaler. I assisted him, nearly beside myself with anxiety, for the strongest influences had been brought to bear upon me to dissuade him from making this attempt. I had been told that one of two things was sure to happen; either the test would fail and my husband would be ruined by the world's ridicule, or he would kill the patient and be tried for manslaughter. Thus, I was drawn in two ways; for while I had unbounded confidence in my husband, it did not seem possible that so young a man could be wiser than the learned and scientific man before whom he proposed to make the demonstration'.

In fact, of course, the experiment, and subsequent more major operations, were carried out successfully and news of 'the most glorious, nay, the most God-like discovery of this or any other age' spread with amazing speed. By December 21, for example, Robert Liston performed the first amputation of leg in Europe under ether anaesthesia at University College Hospital London, exclaiming 'This Yankee dodge, gentlemen, beats mesmerism hollow'.

Sadly, the rest of Morton's life was not a happy one; there were acrimonious claims and counter-claims for priority. He had the satisfaction of using ether with great success during the American Civil War. He died in 1868, aged only 48. The citizens of Boston erected a magnificent monument in his honour, the inscription on which reads:

Inventor and revealer of anaesthetic inhalation
By whom pain in surgery was averted and annulled
Before whom in all time surgery was agony
Since whom science has controlled the pain.

In fact, ether was first used by Crawford Williamson Long (1815–1878) of Jefferson, Georgia, who removed two cysts from the back of the neck of a Mr James Venable in March 1842 and then carried out a number of other operations, including amputation of a toe and fingers with success. However, it was not until 1849, after Long had read the numerous articles on the use of ether in medical journals, that he published his own experiences.

John C Warren "Inhalation of ethereal vapor for the prevention of pain in surgical operations"

Boston Medical and Surgical Journal 1846; 35: 375–379

'Application has been made to me by R H Eddy, Esq in a letter dated 30 November, in behalf Dr W T G Morton, to furnish an account of the operations witnessed and performed by me, wherein his new discovery for preventing pain was employed. Dr M. has also proposed to me to give him the names of such hospitals as I know of in this country, in order that he may present them with the use of his discovery. These applications, and the hope of being useful to my professional brethren, especially those concerned in the hospitals which may have the benefit of Dr M.'s proposal, have induced me to draw up the following statement, and to request that it may be made public through your journal.

The discovery of a mode of preventing pain in surgical operations has been an object of strong desire among surgeons from an early period. In my surgical lectures I have almost annually alluded to it, and stated the means which I have usually adopted for the attainment of this object. I have also freely declared, that notwithstanding the use of very large doses of narcotic substances, this desideratum had never been satisfactorily obtained. The successful use of any article of the materia medica for this purpose, would therefore be hailed to me as an important alleviation to human suffering. I have in consequence readily admitted the trial of plans calculated to accomplish this object, whenever they were free from danger.

About five weeks since, Dr Morton, dentist of this city, informed me that he had invented an apparatus for the inhalation of a vapor, the effect of which was to to produce a state of total insensibility of pain, and that he had employed it successfully in a sufficient number of cases in his practice to justify him in a belief of its efficacy. He wished for an opportunity to test its power in surgical operations, and I agreed to give him such an opportunity as soon as practicable.

Being at that time in attendance as Surgeon of the Massachussetts General Hospital, a patient presented himself in that valuable institution a few days after my conversation with Dr Morton who required an operation for a tumor of the neck, and agreeably to my promise I requested the attendance of Dr M.

On October 16, the patient being prepared for the operation, the apparatus was applied to his mouth by Dr Morton for about three minutes, at the end of which time he sank into a state of insensibility. I immediately made an incision about three inches long through the skin of the neck, and began a dissection among important nerves and blood vessels without any expression of pain on the part of the patient. Soon after he began to speak incoherently, and appeared to be in an agitated state during the remainder of the operation. Being asked immediately afterwards whether he had suffered much, he said that he had felt as if his neck had been scratched; but subsequently, when inquired of by me, his statement was, that he did not experience pain at the time, although aware that the operation was proceeding.

The effect of the gaseous inhalation in neutralizing the sentient faculty was made perfectly distinct to my mind by this experiment, although the patient during a part of its prosecution exhibited appearances indicative of suffering. Dr Morton has apprised me, that the influence of his application would last but a few minutes after its intermission; and as the operation was necessarily protracted, I was not disappointed that its success was only partial.

On the following day, an operation was done by Dr Hayward, on a tumor of the arm, in a female patient at the Hospital. The respiration of the gas was in this case continued during the whole of the operation. There was no

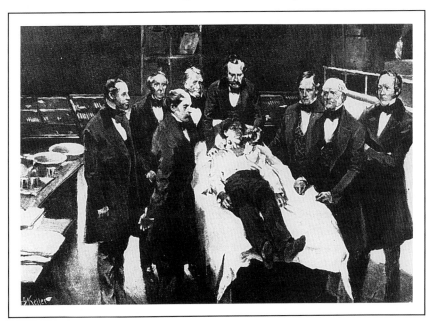

The first operation under general anaesthesia
Courtesy of the Massachusetts General Hospital, Boston

exhibition of pain, excepting some occasional groans during its last stage, which she subsequently stated to have arisen from a disagreeable dream. Noticing the pulse in this patient before and after the operation, I found it to have risen from 80 to 120 . . .

The success of this process in the prevention of pain for a certain period being quite established, I at once conceived it to be my duty to introduce the apparatus into the practice of the Hospital, but was immediately arrested by learning that the proprietor intended to obtain an exclusive patent for its use. It now became a question, whether, in accordance with that elevated principle long since introduced into the medical profession, which forbids its members to conceal any useful discovery, we could continue to encourage an application we were not allowed to use ourselves, and of the components of which we were ignorant. On discussing this matter with Dr Hayward, my colleague in the Hospital, we came to the conclusion, that we were not justified in encouraging the further use of this new invention, until we were better satisfied on these points. Dr Hayward thereupon had a conversation with Dr Morton, in consequence of which Dr M. addressed to me a letter. In this he declared his willingness to make known to us the article employed, and to supply assistance to administer the inhalation whenever called upon. These stipulations he has complied with.

This being done, we thought ourselves justified in inviting Dr Morton to continue his experiments at the Hospital and elsewhere; and he directly after November 7 attended at a painful and protracted operation performed by me, of the excision of a portion of the lower jaw, in which the patient's sufferings were greatly mitigated. On the same day an amputation of the thigh of a young woman was performed at the Hospital by Dr Hayward. In this case the respiration of the ethereal vapor appeared to be entirely successful in preventing the pain of the operation; the patient stating, afterwards, that she did not know that anything had been done to her . . .

The phenomena presented in these operations afford grounds for many interesting reflections, but it being my principal intention at this time to give a simple statement of facts, I shall not pursue the subject further, but close with two or three remarks.

1st. The breathing of the ethereal vapor appears to operate directly on the cerebral system, and the consequent insensibility is proportionate to the degree of cerebal affection.

2nd. Muscular power was for the time suspended in some cases, in others its loss was partial, and in one instance was scarcely sensible. The great relaxation of muscular action produced by a full dose of the application, leads to the hope that it may be employed with advantage in cases of spasmodic affection, both by the surgeon and by the physician.

3rd. The action of the heart is remarkably accelerated in some cases, but not in all.

4th. The respiration is sometimes stertorous, like that of apoplexy.

All these changes soon pass off without leaving any distinct traces behind them, and the ordinary state of the functions returns. This has been the course of things in the cases I have witnessed, but I think it quite probable, that so powerful an agent may sometimes produce other and even alarming effects. I therefore would recommend, that it should never be employed except under the inspection of a judicious and competent person.

Let me conclude by congratulating my professional brethren on the acquisition of a mode of mitigating human suffering, which may become a valuable agent in the hands of careful and well-instructed practitioners, even if it should not prove of such general application as the imagination of sanguine persons would lead them to anticipate.'

References

Long CW. An account of the first use of sulphuric ether by inhalation as an anaesthetic in surgical operations. *Southern Medical and Surgical Journal* 1879; **6**: 705– 713.
MacQuitty B. *The Battle for Oblivion: The Discovery of Anaesthesia.* London: Harrap, 1969.
Scott Earle A. *Surgery in America* 2nd edition, New York: Praegar, 1983.
Warren JC. Inhalation of ethereal vapor for the prevention of pain in surgical operations. *Boston Medical and Surgical Journal* 1846; **35**: 375–379.

[3]

Joseph Lister
The first antiseptic operations (1867)

On August 12th 1865, an operation was performed that was to be the watershed between two eras of surgery, the primitive and the modern. Yet, the operation itself was hardly an operation. There was none of the glamour and ritual of the modern operating theatre; no steely eyes gleaming over white masks, no clink of steel against steel, no rhythmic pumping of elaborate anaesthetic equipment. It was, indeed the dressing and splintage of a compound fracture of the tibia in a young lad aged 11 years named James Greenlees. The surgeon was the 38 year old professor of Surgery at the Glasgow Royal Infirmary, Joseph Lister.

Lister was born in 1827 in the pleasant country property of Upton Park. Today, this is the site of a block of council apartments called Joseph Lister Court in the East End of London. His father was a prosperous Quaker merchant. Joseph studied Medicine at University College, London and

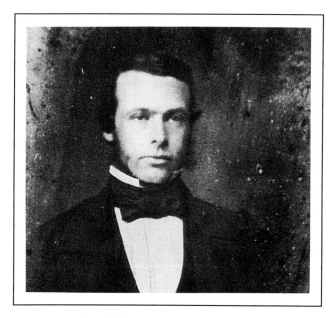

Joseph Lister as a young man
(Reproduced with permission of Dr Gerald Tidy and the
Hertfordshire Medical and Pharmaceutical Museum, Hitchin)

qualified in 1852. The following year, he went to train under James Syme at the Edinburgh Royal Infirmary, married his chief's daughter and was soon elected to the surgical staff. In 1860, Lister was appointed Professor of Surgery in the University of Glasgow and took charge of beds at the Glasgow Royal Infirmary. At that time, Lister, like so many surgeons before him, was puzzled by the observation that a closed fracture, no matter how severe, would heal without infection. In contrast, a compound fracture, complicated by even only a minor puncture wound, would usually suppurate and the victim was lucky to get away with his life, let alone his limb. Indeed, many surgeons would advise immediate amputation in cases where the wound was at all extensive. In some way, exposure of the fracture to air could be lethal. In 1865, the Professor of Chemistry, Thomas Anderson, told Lister of the publications by Louis Pasteur between 1857 and 1860 which proved conclusively that putrefaction was due to bacteria and not merely exposure to air. At once, it became obvious to Lister that

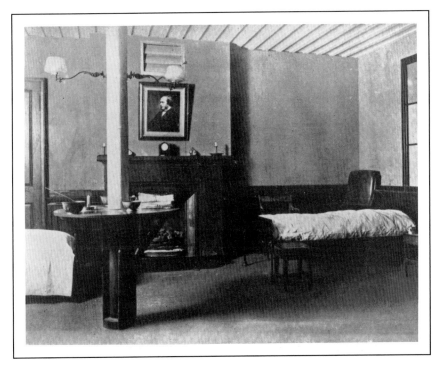

Lister's Male accident ward side room in the Royal Infirmary Glasgow—the scene of his first use of antiseptic surgery
(From D. Guthrie *Lord Lister. His Life and Doctrine*. Edinburgh, Livingstone 1949, reproduced with permission of Churchill-Livingstone)

it was not the air but what it carried into the wound which resulted in the suppuration, pus and gangrene which plagued the surgical wards of those days.

It was clearly impossible to kill microbes in wounds by means of heat, as Pasteur had done in his experiments. Some chemical substance would need to be used. Lister tried a number of different compounds with little success. He then read that carbolic acid had been used with excellent results as a means of purifying the stinking sewage at Carlisle, where it had also been noted that this substance destroyed the microbes which were parasitic on cattle grazing in the neighbouring fields. Lister's first sample was a sticky, smelly fluid, almost insoluble in water but soluble in oil. A purer preparation of carbolic acid was soon obtained and was soluble in 20 parts of water.

The first case in Lister's series, quoted below, was a success. The second case was less happy. This was a 32 year old labourer, whose compound fracture of the leg produced only a small external wound. Identical treatment was employed as in the first patient, and after eleven days progress seemed to be excellent. Lister went off for a short holiday, leaving the house staff in charge. Hospital gangrene developed and the leg had to be amputated. Surgeons should never go on holiday in the middle of an important experiment!

Lister delayed the publication of his results until a total of 11 cases of compound fracture had been managed by the antiseptic technique. There was only one death, the sixth in the series, a 57 year old quarryman with a compound fracture of the thigh as a result of a rock fall. After making good progress for several weeks he died from haemorrhage as a result of perforation of the femoral artery by a sharp fragment of bone. There was the one failure mentioned above and nine successes.

Enormous new vistas of surgery now lay open. Before Lister, surgeons hesitated to inflict an incision through the intact skin because of the extreme risk of wound infection. However, by December 1870, Lister was confident enough to operate on a man with gross malunion of the ulna. The wound healed by first intention. He then performed an open reduction of a fractured patella, daring to open the intact knee joint and to wire the two fragments together; the wound healed. Success followed success as the new antiseptic method became firmly established.

Lister became successively Professor of Surgery in Edinburgh in 1869 and then in 1877 at King's College Hospital in London. In his later years, he was showered with honours, being knighted in 1883 and created a Peer in 1897, the first occasion in which a doctor was promoted to the House of Lords. Lister died in 1912. There is a fine statue in his memory in Portland Place, a short walk from his London home in Park Crescent, just outside Regent's Park in London. It is, as far as I know, the only monument to a surgeon in the United Kingdom, apart from busts to John Hunter in Leicester Square and Lincoln's Inn Fields.

Herewith Lister's first success and first failure of antiseptic surgery:

Joseph Lister "On a new method of treating compound fracture, abscess etc. with observations on the conditions of suppuration"

Lancet 1867; 1: 326

'Case 1. James Greenlees, aged eleven years, was admitted into the Glasgow Royal Infirmary on the 12th August 1865, with compound fracture of the left leg, caused by the wheel of an empty cart passing over the limb a little below its middle. The wound, which was about an inch and a half long, and three quarters of an inch broad, was close to, but not exactly over, the line of fracture of the tibia. A probe, however, could be passed beneath the integument over the seat of fracture and for some inches beyond it. Very little blood had been extravasated into the tissues.

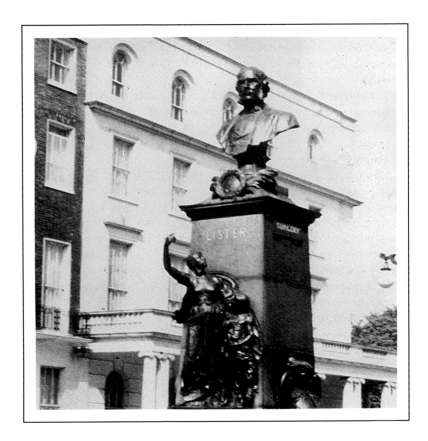

Lister's statue in Park Crescent, London

My house surgeon, Dr Macfee, acting under my instructions, laid a piece of lint dipped in liquid carbolic acid upon the wound, and applied lateral pasteboard splints padded with cotton wool, the limb resting on its outer side, with the knee bent. It was left undisturbed for four days, when, the boy complaining of some uneasiness, I removed the inner splint and examined the wound. It showed no signs of suppuration, but the skin in its immediate vicinity had a slight blush of redness. I now dressed the sore with lint soaked with water having a small proportion of carbolic acid diffused through it; and this was continued for five days, during which the uneasiness and the redness of the skin disappeared, the sore meanwhile furnishing no pus, although some superficial sloughs caused by the acid were separating, but the epidermis being excoriated by the dressing, I substituted for it a solution of one part of carbolic acid in from ten to twenty parts of olive oil, which was used for four days, during which a small amount of imperfect pus was produced from the surface of the sore, but not a drop appeared from beneath the skin. It was now clear that there was no longer any danger of deep-seated suppuration, and simple water dressing was employed. Cicatrization proceeded just as in an ordinary granulating sore. At the expiration of six weeks I examined the condition of the bones, and, finding them firmly united, discarded the splints; and two days later the sore was entirely healed, so that the cure could not be said to have been at all retarded by the circumstance of the fracture being compound.

Certificate of attendance at Lister's surgical lectures 1867–8
(Given to the author by Dr Gerald Tidy, Hitchin)

This, no doubt, was a favourable case, and might have done well under ordinary treatment. But the remarkable retardation of suppuration, and the immediate conversion of the compound fracture into a simple fracture with a superficial sore, were most encouraging facts.

Case 2. Patrick F, a healthy labourer, aged thirty-two, had his right tibia broken on the afternoon of the 11th September 1866, by a horse kicking him with its full force over the anterior edge of the bone about its middle. He was at once taken to the infirmary, where Mr Miller, the house surgeon in charge, found a wound measuring about an inch by a quarter of an inch, from which blood was welling profusely.

He put up the fracture in pasteboard splints, leaving the wound exposed between their anterior edges, and dressing it with a piece of lint dipped in carbolic acid, large enough to overlap the sound skin about a quarter of an inch in every direction. In the evening he changed the lint for another piece, also dipped in carbolic acid, and covered this with oiled paper. I saw the patient next day, and advised the daily application of a bit of lint soaked in carbolic acid over the oiled paper; and this was done for the next five days. On the second day there was an oozing of red fluid from beneath the dressing, but by the third day this had ceased entirely. On the fourth day, when, under ordinary circumstances, suppuration would have made its appearance, the skin had a natural aspect, and there was no increase of swelling, while the uneasiness he had previously felt was almost entirely absent. His pulse was 64, and his appetite improving.

On the seventh day, though his general condition was all that could be wished, he complained again of some uneasiness, and the skin about the still adherent crust of blood, carbolic acid, and lint was found to be vesicated, apparently in consequence of the irritation of the carbolic acid. From the seventh day the crust was left untouched till the eleventh day the entire sore, with the exception of one small spot where the bone was bare, presented a healthy granulating aspect, the formation of pus being limited to the surface of the granulations.

I now had occasion to leave Glasgow for some weeks, and did so feeling that the cure was assured. On my return, however, I was deeply mortified to learn that hospital gangrene attacked the sore soon after I went away, and made such havoc that amputation became necessary.'

References

Fisher RB. *Joseph Lister 1827–1912*. London: Macdonald and Jane's, 1977.
Guthrie D. *Lord Lister. His Life and Doctrine*. Edinburgh: Livingstone, 1949.
Lister J. On a new method of treating compound fracture, abscess etc. with observations on the conditions of suppuration. *Lancet* 1867; **1**: 326.

[4]

Jules Péan

The first successful elective splenectomy (1867)

It is surprising how often a major breakthrough in surgery results from a wrong diagnosis! This is easy enough to understand if we put ourselves in the position of those pioneer surgeons, in the early days of abdominal and pelvic surgery, who had to rely on clinical diagnosis without the benefits of modern radiological imaging. A similar such 'first', the first cholecystotomy for gall stones performed by John Bobbs in 1868, who carried out a laparotomy with the working pre-operative diagnosis of a suspected ovarian cyst, is described in chapter 5.

The first successful elective splenectomy was carried out at an exploratory operation for a suspected ovarian tumour.

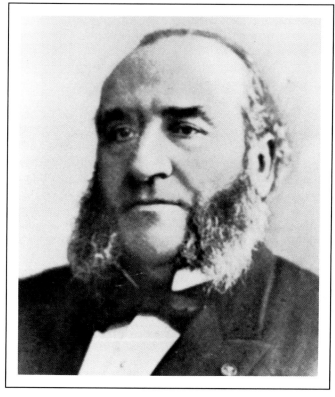

Jules Péan
(Courtesy of Professor Louis Hollender, Strasbourg)

The surgeon was Jules Péan (1830–98), who was the son of a miller and who had to support himself as a medical student in Paris entirely by fees received from coaching his fellow students in Anatomy. After passing out first in the examinations for the election of resident medical officers at the Paris hospitals in 1853, his promotion was rapid and for twenty years he served as surgeon of the St Louis Hospital in Paris. In 1879 he carried out the first gastrectomy for a carcinoma of the stomach but the patient died on the fifth post-operative day. It was not until January 1881 that Theodor Billroth performed the first successful gastric resection in Vienna (Chapter 8).

Péan was a pioneer of vaginal hysterectomy and of laryngectomy. In 1868 he devised forceps for the compression of arteries which incorporated in the handles a ratchet to lock them in position. These were later modified by Spencer Wells, but in France these instruments are still termed 'les pinces de Péan'.

He died suddenly of pneumonia while still busily engaged in his enormous private practice. Undoubtedly he was one of the fathers of modern French surgery.

The following is an abstracted translation of Péan's very detailed case report (translated by H Ellis)

Jules Péan "Splenectomy (ablation of a splenic cyst and complete extirpation of hypertrophied spleen); recovery!"

L'union Medicale 1867; 4:340 and 373

'Mademoiselle Adele Cercily, aged 20 years, of robust constitution and a lymphatic temperament, had enjoyed good health until her first symptoms became manifest two years previously, comprising increase in the volume of the hypogastric region accompanied by pain in this area. The symptoms became worse little by little but two months before the operation her sufferings had become severe . . . and had resisted all medical means of relief.

The patient came to consult me on 20th August; her sufferings had become insupportable so that she was prepared to accept any means of relief.

Here are the results of the examination at that time:
General state profoundly disabled; an advanced degree of anaemia; digestive function profoundly disturbed; dysmenorrhea; respiration a little impaired. The abdomen is increased in size and presents very considerable protusion in hypogastrium. The protrusion, whose surface presented several large bosselations, otherwise resembled, by its position, its extent and its shape, that of a gravid uterus in the last weeks of gestation. The circumference of the abdomen measured 1 metre 10 cms. Palpation produced a little pain in some places; the tumour had a variable consistency, was more firm, solid and resembled that of fibroma.

On percussion, absolute dullness over all the surface of the tumour. Resonance evident over all its surrounds, in the epigastrium, hypogastrium and above all its periphery and in particular on its superior border; it was completely devoid of mobility.

Vaginal examination reveals an intact hymen. The uterus is normal and appears pushed down by the weight of the tumour . . .

On the 6th September, at the Convent of Augustine Sisters, I operated, assisted by Drs Ordonez, Desarénes, Gandin, Morpain, Cossé and Magdelain, an intern on my unit. The patient struggled against the action of the chloroform and it was necessary to stop on several occasions during the course of the operation because of vomiting, which constituted a serious complication. An incision was made along the midline from the umbilicus to the pubis through the layers of the abdominal wall, which were fairly fatty; four ligatures were placed on the divided vessels, the peritoneum was incised over a grooved director and no liquid escaped from the peritoneal cavity.

The edges of the incision having been retracted, the anterior surface of the tumour appeared, tightly pressed against the abdominal wall and covered along its whole extent by the omentum, which was impossible to sweep away because of its adherence and across which I resolved to carry out a puncture with the aid of a large calibre trocar. This puncture produced three litres of thick viscid liquid of yellowish brown colour. The tumour having become diminished in volume, I was able to introduce my hand into the peritoneal cavity and, in palpating inferiorly, it was possible to detach the omentum from the pelvis and the tumour, to both of which it was adherent, this being followed by an effusion of blood, which arrested without it being necessary to apply a ligature.

In vain did I search at the side of the ovary, for the pedicle or the base of the cyst. It was possible for me to establish not only that there was no pedicle but also that the tumour was completely independent in all its inferior portion from the organs contained within the pelvic cavity. Knowing that cysts which resemble those originating in the ovary may develop in the mesentery or in the renal parenchyma, I turned my attention to this possibility, but the results of my examination were completely negative. The impossibility of delivering the tumour for fuller exploration made it necessary to enlarge the incision, which I prolonged on the left side to four finger breadths above the umbilicus. This led me in the superior angle of the incision to that portion of the cyst which constituted a pouch evacuated by the puncture; it still contained liquid. In order to evacuate this completely and to facilitate extraction, the thinnest part of the wall of this pouch was excised and I was able to lift it out.

We were then struck by the appearance of the cyst, its colour, the nature of the tissue which constituted its walls, particularly in those parts which were thickest, and soon no further doubt was possible: the investigation of the points of attachment of the cyst, the manual exploration of the dome of the diaphragm and of the left hypochondrium, which allowed delimitation of the fleshy mass which constituted the superior part of the tumour, all proved that it was the spleen which was involved: the cyst, situated in front and below, was developed in a hypertrophied mass in the thickness of which it occupied a considerable extent.

The cyst was unilocular and its bosselation, as well as differences in the resistance of various parts of its surface, established by palpation, were due to differences in the thickness of the various parts of its walls, the thickness of which varied from a few millimetres up to 4 or 5 cms. The surface of the tumour was furrowed by blood vessels and divided posteriorly by a large venous trunk 1.5 cm in diameter.

In spite of the extent of the incision, the complete extraction of the tumour was rendered impossible because of its situation and I had to think of removing it in pieces.

Considering the disposition of the arterial system of the spleen, which divides into independent segments one from the other, we proceeded with successive ligation of the various branches of the splenic artery to isolate that portion of the spleen which bore the cyst; the large vein on the posterior aspect having previously been tied as close as possible to its entry into the splenic vein, the inferior part of the tumour was resected and this division did not give rise, as we hoped, to any haemorrhage.

The superior part of the tumour, made up of about a third of the total mass of the hypertrophied spleen, was now rendered accessible; several intestinal and omental adhesions were detached which only opened some small vessels, where compression alone sufficed to arrest the bleeding. This is how I proceeded to remove this last portion of the spleen. As a preliminary, four metal ligatures were carefully placed on the gastrosplenic ligament as near as possible to the spleen in the narrow space which separated the tail of the pancreas and the greater curvature of the stomach. These ligatures served to include all the vessels and to remove all risk of haemorrhage. To protect ourselves from any immediate danger, we proceeded to the extirpation of the remaining portions by their successive destruction by means of a hot cautery, after having crushed them in a special clamp. These successive cauterisations reached the highest limits of the substance of the spleen placed below these ligatures so that not a vestige of the splenic tissue remained.

The four metal ligatures were then cut short and left within the abdominal cavity.

The patient did not lose more than 100 g of blood during the operation. During the evacuation of the cyst, none of the fluid was spilled into the abdomen. In spite of this I did not neglect the care which I take in similar cases and having cleaned the loops of intestine, I sponged out the peritoneal cavity several times. I then closed the wound and in order to have a complete closure I inserted nine metal ligatures into the abdominal wall sufficiently far from the lips of the incision and including the parietal peritoneum and five sutures twisted round on the places which gaped between the ligatures.

The operation, thus terminated, had taken a little more than two hours; it had been carried out without notable loss of blood, apart from that which was contained in such an abundance of tissue of such a tumour. During the whole duration of the operation the patient was maintained in a state of perfect insensibility; the chloroforming was so complete that it took nearly half an hour before she emerged from her profound sleep in which she had been artificially immersed.

During the passage of the night which followed the operation there was no fever; the patient did not complain of any malaise and had several vomits due to the effects of the chloroform; she took some cold clear soup and several stimulating drinks.

The next day, the vomiting recurred on a couple of occasions and produced a little pain in the left hypochrondium. All the time the abdomen remained insensitive to pressure and gave no evidence of distension. The pulse was normal at 90 beats.

The third day, the vomiting ceased; the patient regained all her cheerfulness; the relief was such that she was able to sit up and to return to her bed without any pain; the abdomen was supple and not painful on pressure.

The edges of the wounds were perfectly apposed and the pins of the interrupted twisted sutures were removed.

The fifth day, all the metal stitches were removed and replaced by a collodion dressing. At this time the general state of the patient was as satisfactory as if she had not been submitted to an operation; she had neither fever nor pain and her digestive functions were so satisfactory that she was allowed solid food.

From the eighth day, the patient was able to get out of her bed and lie on a chaise longue without any reaction being thus provoked. The healing of the wound was solid and complete throughout its extent.'

References

Ellis H. *The Spleen.* Austin: Silvergirl, 1988.

Péan J. Opération de splenotomie (ablation d'un kyste splénique et extirpation complète de la râte hypertrophée); guerison! *L'Union Medical* 1867; **4**: 340–344 and 373–377.

[5]
John Stough Bobbs
The first cholecystotomy for gall stones (1868)

Gall stones have been found in ancient Egyptian mummies and presumably caused symptoms since the earliest days of mankind. Certainly, 'inflammation of the liver' was well recognized by the Greeks, and described by Paulus Aegineta. Morgagni reported 20 autopsies in which gall stones were found in 1761. Petit in Paris in 1743 described a lady who had her distended gall

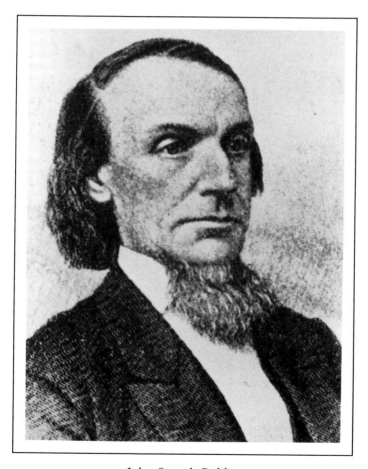

John Stough Bobbs
(From J. O. Robinson *Silvergirl's Surgery—The Biliary Tract* Austin, Silvergirl 1985, reproduced with the author's permission)

bladder drained under the impression that it was an abscess. Several months later, he was able to extract a stone the size of a pigeon's egg from the depths of the persistent fistula.

However, it was an internist who encouraged surgeons to carry out a deliberate operation for gall stones. John Thudichum (1829–1901) was not only a clinician but also lectured on pathological chemistry at St Thomas's Hospital, London and published a treatise on the chemical composition of gall stones. In a paper he published in 1859, he advised that the surgeon could fix the gall bladder to the abdominal wall through a small incision and then, having allowed adhesions to form, could open the gall bladder, extract the stones and the resultant fistula should then heal spontaneously.

However, it was not until 1867 that John Stough Bobbs (1809–1870), Professor of Surgery in the Indiana Central Medical School, who, apparently, was unaware of Thudichum's paper, performed the procedure and published it the following year. The operation was carried out under chloroform in a third floor room above a Drug Store where Bobbs rented a room for his operations. This procedure was performed, of course, without antiseptic precautions—Lister's paper on antisepsis was published in this same year of 1867 (see chapter 3). The pre-operative diagnosis was of a probable ovarian cyst. The patient, apart from her wound infection, made a good recovery and outlived not only Bobbs but also six of the eight medical witnesses of the operation.

The case was reported in the Transactions of the Indiana State Medical Society at its 18th annual session—not a journal that would have been widely read in the USA and certainly not in Europe.

It was not for another decade that further operations to remove stones from the gall bladder were reported by Marion Sims, (who introduced the term 'cholecystotomy') Theodor Kocher in Berne, W. W. Keen in Philadelphia and Lawson Tait in Birmingham. It was only after many years that John Bobbs received the world-wide accolade of a surgical first.

It remained for Carl Langenbuch of Berlin, to perform the first cholecystectomy in 1882 (chapter 9).

Bobbs was a Pennsylvanian of Dutch extraction. He trained at Jefferson Medical College in his home state, and served as a medical officer in the Civil War, where he became an experienced chloroformist. He went on to become foundation Professor of Surgery in Indianapolis.

John S Bobbs, MD "Case of Lithotomy of the gall bladder"

Transactions of the Indiana State Medical Society 1868; 18: 10

'EW aged 30 years, requested my advice by request by Dr Newcomer for an enlargement in the right side. She is of spare habit, medium size, and nervous temperament. Has usually enjoyed pretty good, but never robust health. About four years ago she observed an enlargement in the right iliac region, about the size of a hickory nut. Its position she represented to have been low down in the iliac region. There was no tenderness of the part. Her health at the time was bad, and continued so for several months. She had neuralgia of the stomach, and food and drink created much distress. This was produced by much exercise also, and usually lasted three or four hours. The enlargement continued to increase in size, and became tender after exercise, and ultimately disabled her from walking or, as she expressed it, 'last winter (1867) she could not put her foot to the floor'. Since January 1867, the enlargement has grown faster and given more trouble.

Examination revealed a tumor just inside the right iliac bone, tender to pressure. Its outline could not be well made out, except on the right side, where its boundary was pretty distinctly defined. The most prominent part could be traced on its lower border, while its inner margin, toward the spine, was less distinctly defined, and its upper limits still more obscurely marked. It admitted of a slight degree of motion from side to side and upward, but its movements left it uncertain whether the most prominent portion was the chief part of the enlargement, or only a projection from a deeper seated growth. The walls of the abdomen were tense, and slightly protuberant. The most careful examination per vaginum and otherwise disclosed no connections with the uterus or its appendages, although the limited motion in the parts did not seem to be enlarged, as it could not be felt above the pubis.

The patient was exceedingly anxious to have something done for her relief, as she could not take any exercise, or follow her occupation of running a sewing machine, without its being followed by pain and tenderness of the parts, and which extended down the right limb.

So much obscurity surrounded the case that I requested further examination and consideration at some subsequent period, before attempting to diagnose the character of the tumor. This examination was made but revealed nothing new, and tended to confirm the opinion partially arrived at on the previous occasion, that the enlargement had no connection with the uterine organs but beyond this, nothing definite as to its character or connections could be made out. It had the position and appearance of ovarian tumor, and the patient so regarded it, from the opinion of other physicians whom she consulted. She was informed that its ovarian character was doubtful, and its true nature very uncertain, and if it were the former I could give no assurance that it could be successfully removed. She, however, so persisted in the request that I should undertake its removal, that I finally consented to make the attempt, and on the 15th of June 1867, assisted by Drs Newcomer, Todd, Comingore, Meads, Moore, Avery, and a medical student, proceeded to do so.

An exploratory incision was made between the umbilicus and pubis, the patient being under the influence of chloroform. The omentum was found to be thickened and adherent to the walls of the abdomen. It was separated by a finger, as far as this could reach, towards the right side, along the whole extent of the section—about four inches in length—in hopes of reaching some part where no adhesion existed. Failing in this, with two fingers of either hand the omentum was torn through over the tumor, so as to admit the finger which came upon the protuberant portion of it. Passing the finger around this, some adhesions were broken up, and the tumor traced upward. Other adhesions which it had formed with the parts around it were also discovered, and what seemed to be a smaller lobe in its upper part, but no pedicle or attachment could be felt. Enlarging the opening through the omentum, the tumor was plainly visible, but the orifice would not admit of its exit. The wound through the abdominal walls was carried an inch above the umbilicus on the right side, over the prominent part of the enlargement, which was made to pass through it. This was found to be oval in form, about five inches in length, and two inches in diameter at its widest part, tense, and evidently contained a pellucid fluid. No pedicle could be made out, and the sack showing its contents to be transparent, its lower margin was cut through, when a perfectly limpid fluid escaped, propelling, with considerable force, several solid bodies about the size of ordinary rifle bullets. Introducing the finger other solid bodies were felt, but not in the main sack. A number were hooked out with the finger, and varied in size from that of a mustard seed to that of a bullet. One of the latter size could be distinctly felt, but no communication between the space containing this and the main sack could be found, and it was not removed, being situated at the extreme end of the finger. The sack had the appearance externally of an hydatid, its walls were of the thickness of ordinary cuticle, smooth in its inner aspect, and were whitish and semi-pellucid. Pulling it downward, after being exhausted, brought into plain view the right lobe of the liver, to the lower surface of which it was attached by a broad linear base like the gall bladder. The finger introduced into the sack detected what seemed to be smaller sacculi opening into the main one.

It had the appearance of an enlarged gall bladder, or an appendage to this, although its size, the clear serous character of its contents, and the thickness and semi-transparency of its walls, might justify some degree of doubt upon this subject. From its form, attachments and solid accretions, one of which could be so distinctly felt in a diverticulum but which I did not succeed in removing, seemed to mark its identity with the gall bladder, and deterred me from the excision of the sack, as I should otherwise have done. I therefore put a stitch in the cut lips of its walls and cut the ends closely. The step was suggested by the apprehension that if any portion of its solid contents should have been overlooked, their escape into the cavity of the abdomen would be prevented and the belief that the sack in the event of its refilling with fluid would become adherent to the walls of the abdomen and be within the reach of a trochar and make it practicable to obliterate it by injection if it became necessary.

It would have been gratifying to have determined the condition and relations of the parts more satisfactorily, but the adhesions existing, as the result of past peritoneal inflammation, rendered this impracticable without increased hazard to the patient.

The wound was closed by sutures and adhesive plaster, no vessel requiring to be ligated, and thirty drops of laudanum given after the patient was placed in bed.

16th. 8 o'clock, A.M. The patient was slightly feverish; had slept half the night; complained of some soreness on both sides under the ribs. The abdomen very slightly swollen on the right side, which was tender to pressure. Urine was removed by the catheter, as it had been the previous evening. Ordered all company to be excluded, great quietude, and no more movement in bed to be allowed than became necessary to relieve her posture when it became irksome. As she complained of her bed another was placed along side of it upon which she was removed.

17th. Somewhat feverish: pulse 100. Slept some last night; drank some lemonade. Complains that the laudanum made her sick. Tastes bad. Lies on either side or back. No increased fullness of the abdomen. Wound uniting.

Evening. No fever; skin moist. Is very cheerful. Urine drawn off, although she desires to arise and pass it.

18th. Complains of some general soreness and chilliness. Lay at an open window after a rain storm, and she thinks she took cold; the weather having become suddenly cool after being very warm. Ate an egg for breakfast and some rice for dinner, which tasted better than anything taken since the operation. Pulse 95, and full. Can lie on either side or back. Thinks she is not quite so well. Abdomen less full and tender to pressure.

19th. Morning—Is comfortable, except for dysuria. Have not permitted her to rise as she requested, the catheter having been used twice a day since the operation. Is subject to trouble about the bladder, and was much annoyed with it before the operation, being compelled to pass urine at short intervals. Did not think this of sufficient importance to make it known before the operation. Pulse quiet. No fever. Took some breakfast, which relished better than usual.

Evening—Began to complain of the bladder soon after morning visit, when I drew off half a pint of urine. This continued all day, and at 5 o'clock she got partly out of bed and passed some urine. Can never pass urine unless in an upright position. Pulse some disturbed, being 110. Skin warm, but not hot. No fullness of the abdomen. Complains of pain in the left side under the short ribs. No increased tenderness of the abdomen. Passed but little urine when up. Constitutional disturbances more marked than at any time since the day after the operation, but not very marked. Ordered: Bicarbonate soda gr.v. Bi-meconate of morph. gr. 1–10, to be repeated every two hours until relieved. Also, 25 drops of laudanum to be added if necessary after the first portion. Fomentations to the abdomen.

20th. Morning—removed half a pint of urine, which gave much relief. She slept part of the night. Pulse 110. Some fever. Tongue sticky, which she charges to the laudanum taken. No fullness of abdomen or increased tenderness. Complains of pain on the left side, under the ribs. Thinks she cannot move herself so easily. Can lie on either side, but best on the right, but lies mostly on her back, with the knees drawn up. Took a cup of tea.

Evening—is a little feverish; pulse 110. Drew off half a pint of moderately high colored urine. She ate a few strawberries, a slice of bread, and drank a cup of tea at noon. The wound looks closed, the ligatures and plasters not having been disturbed. During the previous night had taken three portions of soda and morphia, and once 30 drops of laudanum, which have been obvious in the quieting influence during the day. One portion of the former was given at noon, and another ordered to be given at night, with the laudanum in addition, if necessary to secure quietude. The bowels having been well evacuated before the operation have not acted since. Fomentations to the abdomen to be continued.

21st. Morning—removed half a pint of high colored urine with much relief. Took one portion of soda and morphia during the night. Slept some; pulse 110. Skin warm, but perspirable. No tumidity of the abdomen, and less tenderness. Mouth sticky from effects of laudanum. Drank a cup of tea.

Evening.—complained from 12 o'clock, of disposition to urinate, which gives her much distress. Removed half a pint of high colored urine. Has taken three portions of the solution of soda and morphia during the day. The pulse is some excited, and skin warm. No tumidity of the abdomen. A healthy discharge is issuing from one point in the wound. No increased tenderness of the abdomen. Ordered the soda and morphia to be continued when required.

22nd. Morning—rested last night after taking two portions of solution and 25 drops of laudanum. Removed half a pint of high colored urine with alkaline smell and some turbidness. Pulse 100. Skin warm and moist. Tongue slightly coated, and mouth pasty. Removed the dressings and stitches from the wound and replaced adhesive straps. The wound was adherent in most of its extent. Some thick pus issued from one point, at the junction of the lower with the middle third of the wound. Abdomen less full and much less tender. Feels much better, and complains of nothing but urinary trouble. Allowed her clothing to be changed, which she has begged permission to do for several days.

From this period her recovery was progressive, and requires no special remark. In about two weeks she was permitted to sit up, and in three weeks to move about her room, and in four to ride out.

Careful examination of the solid concretions removed leaves no doubt of their being biliary calculi. They are irregularly spherical in shape, smooth on the surface which is of a mahogany color, and polished. The interior is of a whitish yellow, striated and porous. They are of light specific gravity, and numbered some forty or fifty, the majority being of the size of small shot. When access to the enlargement was reached, the surrounding parts were so agglutinated by old adhesions as to prevent a satisfactory inspection of its deeper portion. After the sack was opened more space was obtained, and its attachment to the under surface of the liver could be both seen and felt, and had the appearance of an hypertrophied gall bladder. Its lower extremity projected about five inches from the free margin of the liver. The cystic duct was probably obliterated from irritation produced by these concretions, and the one felt at the extremity of the finger was probably lodged in one of the biliary ducts.

Various authors have reported cases of hypertrophy of the gall bladder, but I believe they have usually found traces of healthy or vitiated biliary matter in the fluids contained in the cysts. In this instance the fluid was perfectly pellucid and watery, the solid and coloring matters having either been appropiated by the concretions, or had become absorbed or diffused. The patient's complexion was somewhat sallow, but no more so than is frequently observable in those suffering from organic disease. She was rather anemic.

Since the operation she has had intermittent fever at intervals, and impaired digestion, and at such invasions complains of pain in the region of the enlargement. At other times she suffers no inconvenience, and is able to pursue her calling of working a sewing machine. No appearance of the enlargement recurring is observable, up to the present, ten months since the operation.'

References

Bobbs JS. Case of lithotomy of the gall bladder. *Transactions of the Indiana State Medical Society* 1868; **18**: 10.

Robinson JO. *Biliary Tract*. Austin: Texas. Silvergirl, 1985.

[6]
Jonathan Hutchinson
The first successful operation for intussusception in an infant (1874)

Because of its vivid manifestations of blood-stained mucus passed per rectum, a palpable abdominal mass and, in late cases, a prolapsing mass to be felt in the rectum or even to be seen extruding through the anal verge, it is not surprising that intussusception was one of the earliest forms of intestinal

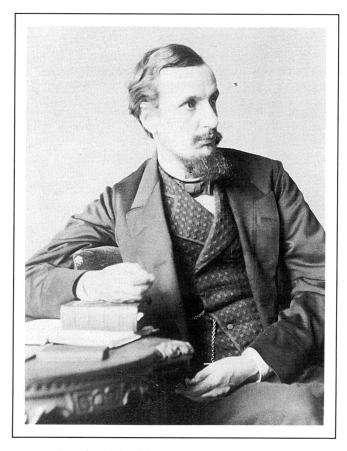

Jonathan Hutchinson as a young surgeon
(Reproduced by permission of the President and Council of the
Royal College of Surgeons of England)

obstruction to be clearly differentiated. Treatment was expectant, with efforts to reduce the intussusception by enemas or by the passage of rectal bougies. Surgeons were encouraged to continue these efforts by occasional reports of successes and by still rarer examples where spontaneous cure resulted from the passage per rectum of the gangrenous segment of strangulated bowel.

The first successful operation for the reduction of an intussusception in an infant was performed in 1871 by Jonathan Hutchinson, who published a detailed report of the case in 1874. In this paper he meticulously tabulated 131 previous case reports.

Jonathan Hutchinson was born in 1828 in Yorkshire of a prosperous Quaker family. He qualified at St Bartholomew's Hospital, London in 1850 and was appointed to the surgical staff of the London Hospital ten years later. He also had appointments to the Hospital for Diseases of the Skin, Moorfields Eye Hospital, the Lock Hospital Blackfriars, the City of London Hospital for Diseases of the Chest and the Liverpool Street Chest Clinic.

He was a man of tremendous industry, a brilliant lecturer and, (as will be illustrated by the following case report), a lucid writer. As well as his interest in abdominal emergency surgery, he made remarkable observations in his other fields of interest, ophthalmology, dermatology and venereal diseases.

Hutchinson was a remarkable clinical observer. This is exemplified by his description of the stigmata of congenital syphilis, which included the pegtop incisor teeth (now known the world over as Hutchinson's teeth), interstitial keratitis and labyrinthine deafness. This grouping of three abnormalities became termed 'Hutchinson's triad'. In 1865 he won the Astley Cooper Prize for an essay on 'Injuries of the Head and their Treatment', in which he described the original observation that in extradural haemorrhage, as the compression of the brain increases, the pupil of the same side undergoes increasing dilatation and becomes increasingly inactive to a bright light. This phenomenon is due to compression of the oculomotor nerve against the tentorium cerebelli (Hutchinson's pupils). He also had a vivid way of describing physical signs; for example, the apple-jelly appearance of some forms of lupus and the 'potato tumour' of the carotid body. He described the mask-like facial appearance of tabes dorsalis (Hutchinson's facies).

His contributions to dermatology, as listed by Russell, were descriptions of arsenical zoster, cheiropompholyx, varicella gangrenosa, summer prurigo, dermatitis gangrenosa infantum, melanotic whitlow, arsenical keratosis, atrophic balanitis, infective angioma (angioma serpiginosum) and solid oedema of the face following recurrent lymphangitis.

Hutchinson wrote numerous books and published ten volumes of *Archives of Surgery* in periodical form between 1889 and 1900; the entire contents of these volumes were written by himself! In the seventh volume of his Archives (1896) is a remarkable report and illustration of identical twin sisters, aged nine, who, at the age of three had developed identical black pigment spots on their lips and inside the mouth. In 1919, Parkes-Weber noted a follow-up on these girls, one of them whom had died following an operation for intussusception 11 years after Hutchinson's original observation. Perhaps Hutchinson's name should be attached eponymously to the syndrome described by Peutz (1921) and by Jeghers and his colleagues in 1949.

In addition to his professional teaching, Hutchinson was a pioneer of science education to the public. In 1890 he established an educational museum and library of natural history near his country home at Haslemere. This was situated in a series of sheds and here he gave regular lectures to the lay public. The subjects ranged from geology, shells, the elephant's skull, lizards, birds and kangaroos to the lives and works of Milton, Wordsworth, Keats and Dürer. He extended these activities in 1898, when he purchased the public rooms at Selby, his birth-place in Yorkshire. Here he established a second museum and travelled up from London to lecture there over the next seven years. Some of his subjects, such as 'life, death and immortality', clashed with the views of some of the local churchmen. Hutchinson supplemented his public lectures with the publication of a monthly journal,

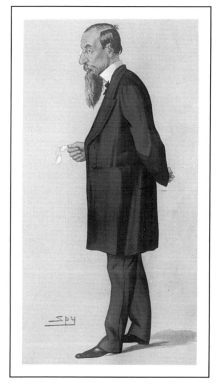

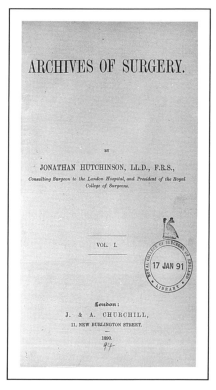

Jonathan Hutchinson in his maturity (Cartoon by 'Spy')

Cover of Vol. 1 of *Archives of Surgery* published by Hutchinson between 1889 and 1900 mostly written by himself, which covered a wide variety of topics in science and literature. His museum at Selby closed after his death. The Haslemere museum, now on its third site, flourishes to this day.

Hutchinson's long association with the Royal College of Surgeons of England started with his election to Council in 1879. He was Hunterian Professor 1879–83, a member of the Court of examiners between 1880 and 1887 and gave the Bradshaw Lecture in 1888, his subject being 'Museums in their relation to medical education'. He served as President in 1889, but resigned after only one year in office; he was probably too much of a reformer for his colleagues on Council. To serve the customary full term of three years as President carried with it a baronetcy on retirement, which he obviously sacrificed. It is known that he refused a peerage offered him by Asquith and only accepted a knighthood in his old age in 1908 in deference to the opinion of his friends, who persuaded him it would be in the interests of science.

In 1911 Hutchinson retired from London and ceased to lecture. He died in his sleep a month before his 85th birthday and was buried beside his wife in Haslemere churchyard. At his request, he had carved on his tombstone the words: 'A man of Hope and Forward-Looking Mind'.

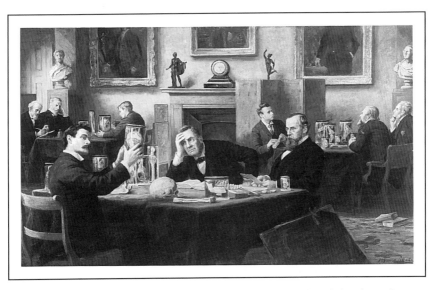

Jonathan Hutchinson examining in the FRCS (the right of the three figures at the foreground table). This painting hangs in the entrance hall of the Royal College of Surgeons of England

Reproduced by permission of the President and Council of the Royal College of Surgeons

Jonathan Hutchinson "A successful case of abdominal section for intussusception: with remarks on this and other methods of treatment"

Transactions of the Medico-Chirurgical Society of London 1874: 57: 31–75

'The case of intussusception which I am about to describe came under my care at the London Hospital in 1871.

The patient was a somewhat delicate female child aged two years. She had previously been seen by my colleague Mr Waren Tay, who had diagnosed her disease and by whom she was transferred to my care in order that she might be admitted as an in-patient.

From her anus there protuded a portion of bowel about two inches long, deeply congested and much swollen. By the side of this the finger could be passed, its full length, into the rectum without reaching the point at which the intussusception began. On carefully examining the extremity of the protruded part, I noticed that it did not present merely a rounded opening as usual in such cases. I was able to identify the pouch and the valve of the caecum, with the opening into the ileum. Of these parts it was of course the mucous membrane which was visible, and the appendix caeci was wholly concealed between the folds of the intussusception. This discovery rendered it evident that we had to deal with an involution of bowel of very unusual length, which commencing at the caecum had allowed the ileum to pass through the entire length of the colon, and actually to become extruded at the anus.

On examination of the child's abdomen externally the tract of bowel involved could be felt like a long firm sausage passing down the left side.

The mother of the child gave us the history that the latter had begun to suffer from pains in the abdomen, rather suddenly, about a month previously. Her first attack of pain was one Sunday afternoon and was such as to cause screaming. It was quickly followed by a motion which contained blood and by frequent vomiting. A fortnight after this the child having been ailing the whole time a protrusion of bowel was noticed at the anus. This was reduced by the surgeon then in attendance and a cork pad was fitted over it. It was found impossible, however, to prevent the prolapse from recurring and the child continued to be sick and to pass blood-stained mucus.

Three days before admission the prolapse increased to such a size that the parents were unable to reduce it and were obliged on three occasions to call in surgical aid for that purpose. There had been no real obstruction of the bowels, but only temporary constipation at times.

The child, at the time of her admission, looked very ill. Her countenance was pale and anxious, and from her mother's description it was evident that her strength had been failing rapidly during the last few days.

It appeared that she was almost constantly engaged in straining to get rid of the bowel which filled the rectum.

Our first measure of treatment consisted in putting the child under chloroform and then whilst she was half up by the feet distending the rectum to the utmost with warm water. By this means the involuted part could be forced up into the abdomen so as to be quite out of reach of the finger, and once or twice I tried to hope that reduction had been effected. On each occasion, however, when the lower bowel was allowed to empty itself, the intussuscepted part became prolapsed as before, and showed clearly that we had gained nothing.

My experience of several other somewhat similar cases, all of which had resulted in death, after patient and repeated attempts by the injection plan, did not encourage me to expect success in this.

It was very evident, from the child's condition, that unless relief were afforded she would not live long, and I therefore felt justified in telling the parents that although an operation would be, in itself very dangerous, yet I thought that it afforded the only chance.

They begged me to give the child a chance if I thought it was one, and we accordingly determined to lose no time.

The child having been taken up into the operation theatre, chloroform was again administered, and I then opened the abdomen in the median line below the umbilicus, and to an extent admitting of the easy introduction of two or three fingers. I now very readily drew out of the wound the intussuscepted mass, which was about six inches long. I found that the serous surfaces did not adhere, and that there was no difficulty whatever in drawing the intussuscepted part out of that into which it had passed. Just as the reduction was finished the appendix caeci made its appearance, confirming the opinion which had been formed as to the precise part of the bowel involved. The opposed serous surfaces did not present a single flake of lymph, and they were congested in only a moderate degree.

Having completed the reduction, I put the bowel back into the abdomen, and closed the wound with harelip pins and interrupted sutures.

The operation had been an extremely simple one, and had not occupied more than two or three minutes.

The abdomen having been well supported by strapping, cotton wool, and a flannel bandage, the child was returned to bed.

The after-treatment consisted in the use of milk enemata every three hours, with the occasional addition of five minims of tincture of opium.

No vomiting occurred after the operation. No food whatever was allowed to be taken by the mouth during the next two days. The temperature on the evening of the operation, was 100.5°, but subsequently fell to 99°, and with the exception of the fifth day, on the evening of which it rose to 101.7°, it never exceeded 100°. Chloroform was administered on two or three occasions to allow of the wound being dressed without the child screaming. The pins were taken out on the fourth day, that is, seventy-two hours after the operation.

I had felt much anxiety as to the healing of the abdominal wound on account of the thinness of the parietes, but nothing untoward occurred.

The child recovered without having ever showed the slightest symptom of peritonitis, and left the hospital in excellent health about three weeks after the operation.'

References

Ellis H. Jonathan Hutchinson (1829–1913). *Journal of Medical Biography* 1993; 1: 11–16.

Hutchinson J. A successful case of abdominal section of intussusception. *Transactions of the Medical Chirurgical Society (London)* 1874; 57: 31–75.

Hutchinson J. Pigmentation of lips and mouth. *Archives of Surgery (London)* 1896; 7: 290.

Russell BF. Dermatology at the London Hospital. *British Journal of Dermatology* 1969; 81: 780–5.

[7]

Sir William Macewen

The first successful excision of an intracranial tumour (1879)

Most neurosurgeons, asked to name the surgeon who performed the first successful excision of an intracranial tumour, are likely to reply, (if reply at all!), Hughes Bennett, who removed a glioma from the cerebral cortex of a man aged 25 after its accurate clinical localization by Rickman Godlee

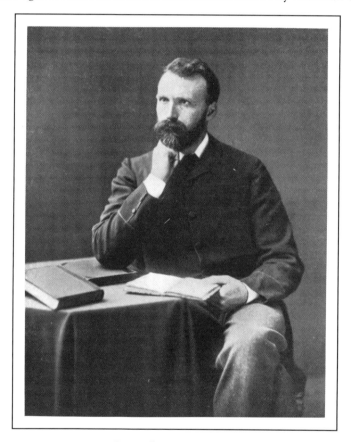

Sir William Macewen
(From JD Comrie *History of Scottish Medicine* published for the
Wellcome Historical Medical Museum by Baillière Tindall and Cox
London 1932. Permission of the Wellcome Institute, London)

(Bennett and Godlee 1884). In fact, five years before this, in 1879, William Macewen had accurately localized and successfully removed what was obviously a meningioma in a girl of 14.

Macewen was undoubtedly the greatest surgical product of the proud and ancient Glasgow Medical School. He was born in 1848 on the Island of Bute on the West Coast of Scotland, the son of a seafaring trader. His education and his whole clinical career was spent in the city of Glasgow. As a medical student, he fell under the influence of Joseph Lister, who left Glasgow to take up the Chair of Surgery at Edinburgh 1869, the year that Macewen qualified. Macewen was an early disciple of Lister, but rapidly advanced the Listerian technique and was one of the early pioneers of aseptic Surgery. Among other innovations, he introduced the sterilizable surgical gown.

He became Regius Professor of Surgery in Glasgow in 1892, occupying the post which Lister had held when Macewen was a student. Interestingly enough, only three years before, Macewen had been offered the Chair of Surgery at the newly established Johns Hopkins Medical School, the reason for his refusal being that he could not be assured that he would be responsible for the supervision and training of the nurses. One wonders what the subsequent history of the Baltimore School of Neurosurgery might have been with Macewen as its chief!

Among his achievements might be mentioned the Macewen osteotomy, for the treatment of genu valgum and valgus, advances in bone grafting, tracheal intubation, the surgery of mastoid infection, the treatment of aneurysm and the first successful pneumonectomy for tuberculosis, which he performed as far back as 1895.

However, Macewen's greatest claim to fame must be as one of the founding fathers of neurosurgery. In 1876 he diagnosed a cerebral abscess in the left frontal lobe of a boy of 11 and advised surgery. This was refused, but at autopsy the diagnosis and localization were brilliantly confirmed. Three years later, the same year that he performed his successful excision of a meningioma, he accurately localized and successfully evacuated a subdural haematoma. By 1893, Macewen had operated upon 24 cases of cerebral abscess with no less than 23 recoveries; a marvellous record, which could hardly be equalled today. Macewen died of pneumonia in 1924. Harvey Cushing wrote, 'To Macewen belongs the distinction of having been the chief pioneer in craniocerebral surgery'.

The following case, therefore, is a worthy landmark in the history of neurosurgery.

W Macewen "Tumour of the Dura Mater—convulsions— removal of tumour by trephining—recovery"

Glasgow Medical Journal 1879; 12: 210–12.

'BW, age 14, was admitted to Ward XXII, 21st June, 1879, suffering from a swelling over the left eye. She had been admitted about a year ago with a supra-orbital periosteal tumour, which was removed. She then enjoyed good health for about three months, when she began to complain of pain over the front and left side of the brow, and about six months ago a tumour was again observed in the old place. Coincidentally with its formation, the pain in front of the head increased. She visited the wards several times as an out patient, and under iodide of potassium, the pain appeared to abate considerably although the tumour continued to increase. It was therefore resolved to bring her into the house and remove the tumour. On admission there was slight contraction of the left pupil, and it responded imperfectly to light. There was a slight prominence on the brow, about the size of a large pea, which seemed to be connected with the periosteum, and which was thought to be of the same character as the supra-orbital tumour; the latter was slightly movable, while the pea-like node was fixed. 27th July, 11 pm—this afternoon, patient was suddenly seized with a convulsion, which was at first confined to the right side of the face and to the right arm. The muscles to the right side of the face were affected by tonic spasm, and the right arm was firmly flexed and violently twitched. A second convulsion followed after an interval of ten minutes, succeeded by others at rapidly diminishing intervals, until, at seven o'clock, they were almost continuous, and extended over the whole body, although the right side was throughout most severely affected. Very soon the face became livid, the respirations fell to only two in the minute, and the pulse, which had been for some time feeble and rather slow, became almost imperceptible. Dr Macewen, who had been noting the progress of the case since the beginning of the attack, concluded that the convulsions depended on pressure on the brain on the left side, in connection somehow with the tumours above noted. He determined therefore to trephine, more especially as a fatal termination of the case seemed imminent. The pea-like node was selected for operation in the first instance. On cutting through the node by a crucial incision, it was found to resemble the usual fungous tumour of the dura mater, and to extend over the frontal bone in a flattened form, apparently connected with the periosteum. The bone underneath was slightly roughened, and imparted a softer feeling to the finger than normal. A trephine an inch in diameter was chosen, and that portion of the bone elevated. The bone was found to be much thickened, and attached to its under surface there was a tumour similar in consistence to that on the outside. The tumour was also seen to be adhering to the inner surface of the skull, while a considerable portion of it was spread over the dura mater. All of this was removed as far as practicable. As the wound was open, the supra-orbital tumour was looked to, and found to be continuous with the node on the frontal bone. The whole mass extended far into the orbital cavity, and this, along with a superficial portion lying under the scalp, was removed. The flaps were then brought together, and horse hair drains left in. The whole operation was performed antiseptically.

July 28—this morning the temperature was 99.2°F, and the patient was perfectly conscious. She answered intelligently, and raised her head to be dressed when desired. There was no return of the convulsions, and she stated that she felt well. Patient has been intelligent throughout the day, and has asked for drinks, etc. She has vomited once. July 30—patient continues to improve, takes an interest in what is going on in the ward, and has asked for solid food. The pupils are now equal. Wound has been dressed daily since the operation. August 1—since yesterday morning, the temperature has been gradually rising till, at 10 pm it reached 102°F. The wound was dressed at 9 pm and immediately afterwards aphasia came on; and, at 11.25 pm convulsions, similar to those which preceded the operation set in. During the day the pupils had been slightly unequal. Bowels were freely moved. August 2, 2 am—convulsions continuous. Temperature 104.6°F. 4 am—convulsions almost subsided, but patient still unconscious. Temperature 105.6°F. 6 am—patient slightly conscious. Temperature 99.6°F. 9 am—head dressed. Patient still aphasic, but more conscious. Power of right arm much impaired. Temperature 98.8°F. 10 pm—has improved considerably during the day. Consciousness almost normal and aphasia gradually disappearing. Temperature 98°F. August 3—patient had a good night. Moves right arm better. Temperature 98°F. 10 pm—patient improving in every respect. Dr Macewen proposes to leave the wound open (but still treated antiseptically), so as to allow it to granulate from the bottom. This will serve two purposes—first, all the pus will have free vent, and, secondly, the aperture will leave room for surgical interference should that be necessary afterwards.

August 7—wound looking very well; perfectly antiseptic, the discharge being very small in quantity, and quite sweet. Temperature since 3rd August has, with very small variations, continued normal.

August 9—wound is gradually filling up. There has been no recurrence of convulsions since the night of 31st July. Patient is allowed to have some solid food; her appetite is good, and she is cheerful and looking well. Wound is now dressed only every second day. Iodide of potassium is still given thrice daily. There is no evidence of any recurrence of the tumour. Temperature normal.

August 15—patient going on very well indeed. Her appetite is good, and she is daily gaining strength.'

References

Bennett AH, Godlee RJ. Excision of a tumour from the brain. Lancet 1884; ii 1090–1.
Bowman AK. *Sir William Macewen A Chapter in the History of Surgery*. London: Hodge, 1942.
Macewen W. Tumour of the dura mater. *Glasgow Medical Journal* 1879; **12**: 210–12.

[8]
Theodor Billroth
The first successful gastrectomy (1881)

It is not often that a single case report—no matter how interesting—actually forms a distinct landmark in surgical history. The report of the successful use of ether by Morton at the Massachusetts General Hospital in 1846 (see chapter 2) certainly sent a shock wave reverberating around the civilized world. In recent years, the example that immediately comes to mind was the first human heart transplant performed by Barnard in Cape Town in 1967.

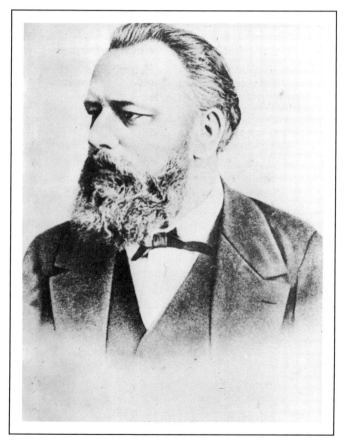

Theodor Billroth
(From H. Ellis *Famous Operations* Media, Harwal 1983)

Partial gastrectomy for gastric cancer had been carried out by Jules Péan in Paris in 1879 but his patient died on the 5th day. A second attempt, with death only 12 hours post-operatively, was made by the Polish surgeon, Ludwig Rydigier, the following year. However, the news that a successful partial gastrectomy had been performed by Theodor Billroth on January 29 1881 at the Allgemeine Krankenhaus in Vienna served as an immense stimulus to the surgery of the alimentary tract, which blossomed rapidly from that date. It is interesting, in passing, that Billroth was aware of Péan's operation but at the time of his own successful case, had not yet learned of Rydigier's operation.

Theodor Billroth was one of the great surgical giants of all time. Qualifying at the University of Berlin, he trained under Bernard Von Langenbeck. At the age of 31 he became Professor of Surgery at Zurich before taking up his appointment in Vienna seven years later. Here, Billroth founded one of the greatest schools of surgery, where he carried out pioneer work in experimental studies, surgical pathology and operative surgery. He pioneered excision of bladder cancer and tumours of the bowel, performed a hindquarter amputation and, in all, personally performed 34 resections of the stomach for cancer. He founded the modern concept of reporting the total clinical experience of a department including operative mortality, complications and five year follow up. However, he sounded a warning note:

'Statistics are like women' he wrote, 'Mirrors of purest virtue and truth or like whores, to use as one pleases!'.

Among Billroth's protegés are included Vincenz Czerny, who became Professor of Surgery in Heidelberg, Carl Gussenbauer, who succeeded Billroth to his chair in Vienna and Johann Von Mikulicz, who became Professor of Surgery in Breslau. Mikulicz developed techniques of pyloroplasty, colectomy and thyroidectomy, pioneered gastroscopy and introduced the surgical mask. Anton Wölfler, a Czech and the first assistant at the time of Billroth's early gastrectomies, pioneered gastroenterostomy and became Professor of Surgery in Prague. Anton Von Eiselberg, Billroth's last great pupil, became Professor of the First Surgical Service in Vienna. Himself a great teacher, he produced no less than 19 chiefs of surgical departments.

Billroth based his surgical advances on sound laboratory studies. Before his successful gastrectomy he had his assistants Gussenbauer and Winiwater work out the technical details of the procedure in the animal laboratory. Billroth wrote 'No insurmountable obstacles to partial excision of the stomach exist either on anatomical, physiological or operative grounds. It must succeed'.

But there was another facet to this surgical giant, perhaps less well known, his life-long association with music. Billroth was born in 1829 in the small fishing village of Bergen on the island of Rügen, off the Baltic shore of Germany. His father was a Lutheran pastor. As a student, his only talent was for music, which he wished to pursue professionally. However, his widowed mother insisted that he study medicine, although he continued to play the piano and to compose.

In Zurich, Billroth first became friendly with Johannes Brahms and this continued when both lived in Vienna. Nearly all Brahms' compositions were first tried out at the home of Billroth. Who knows what he might have achieved if his mother had not made him study medicine!

Billroth died of heart failure in 1894. He was buried in the Cental Cemetery in Vienna, not far from the graves of Beethoven and Schubert and the monument to Mozart.

The report of Billroth's first gastrectomy appears as an open letter to the editor of the *Weiner Meziniche Wochenschrift*. It is dated February 4th and was published a mere seven days after the operation.

Billroth T "Open letter to Dr L Wittelshöfer"

Wiener Medizinische Wochenschrift 1881; 31: 162

'Vienna, 4th February 1881

Dear Colleague

I willingly accede to your request for information about the resection of the stomach which I carried out on January 29th this year, since it concerns the very important question whether it is possible to cure that very common disease, carcinoma of the stomach, by surgical intervention.

Seventy years have passed since a young physician, Karl Theodor Merrem, published a dissertation in which he demonstrated, by means of experiments on dogs, that the pylorus could be excised and the stomach joined to the duodenum, and that two out of three dogs survived the operation. He was bold enough to suggest that this operation should also be performed in human beings with incurable pyloric carcinoma . . . The problem of the best method of closing gastric and intestinal wounds had occupied surgeons for a long time, and arose again and again. The most prominent French, English, and German surgeons have studied this question in the present century, and after Lembert had discovered the only correct principle for such operations (accurate apposition and union of serous surfaces) there were increasingly frequent reports of successful intestinal sutures of accidental wounds. It was, of course, a long time before surgeons ventured to excise diseased segments of the intestines. New and assured progress in this direction was not made until the last decade. In 1871 I pointed out that sections of the oesophagus could be removed in large dogs and that the oesophagus then healed well, leaving a slight, easily dilatable stricture. Czerny was the first to perform this operation successfully in man. Then followed Czerny's experiments on excision of the larynx, after which a few years ago, I successfully removed a human larynx filled with cancerous growths. Then came the experiments of Gussenbauer and Al. v. Winiwarter on the resection of pieces of stomach and intestine, which were subsequently confirmed and extended by Czerny and Kaiser. Martini's and Gussenbauer's success with resection of the sigmoid and mine with gastrorrhaphy (1877) showed that further progress was possible in this direction. The latter operation removed our fears that the scar in the stomach would be digested again by the gastric juice, so I concluded my report on this operation with the words: 'There remains only one bold stride between this operation and resection of a carcinomatous segment of the stomach.'

All this for the reassurance of those who think that the present operation is a foolhardy experiment on man. There is no question of this. Gastric resection, like any other operation, has been fully prepared anatomically, physiologically and technically by my pupils and by myself. Every surgeon who has any personal experience of these animal experiments and similar operations on man becomes convinced that gastric resection is bound to succeed.

This conclusion was also reached by Péan, the Parisian surgeon with the greatest experience of laparotomies. In 1879 he resected 6 cm of carcinomatous pylorus of a patient already exhausted by the disease, who died on the 4th day after the operation. His operative technique, and especially his suture material (catgut), seem to me to have been unfortunately chosen, so I cannot attach much importance to this failure. The operation does not seem to have encouraged Péan very much or he would probably have repeated it, which as far as I know, he has not done, nor has any other surgeon, to my knowledge, ventured to perform this not altogether easy operation.

Only last week a woman with an undoubtedly mobile pyloric carcinoma was brought to me by one of my clinical assistants, Dr Wölfler. After a few days' observation and repeated examination I decided on operation, with the patient's consent, since she felt that in view of her increasing exhaustion and inability to keep her food down, her end was approaching.

This woman of 43 years, always pale, but formerly healthy and well-nourished, mother of 8 living children, fell ill, apparently rather suddenly, with vomiting. All the symptoms of pyloric cancer soon developed, with pyloric stenosis. These being well-known, I shall not repeat them. Masses resembling coffee-grounds were vomited only a few times, and the extreme pallor and emaciation of the woman, as well as the small, rapid pulse had developed only in the last six weeks, after the constant vomiting and the small intake of food. The only food she could keep down for a time, which saved her from starvation, was sour milk.

Preparation for the operation consisted in accustoming her to peptone enemas and gastric irrigation by the usual methods of injection and pumping. In view of the patient's great weakness and the probably long duration of the operation (it had taken Péan 2½ hours). I asked one of my experienced private Assistants, Dr Barbieri, to take charge of the anaesthesia. You will understand that it was necessary for me to devote myself to the operation itself, with no need to worry about anaesthesia. The theatre specially equipped for laparotomies, was, for well-known reasons, heated to 24°. All my

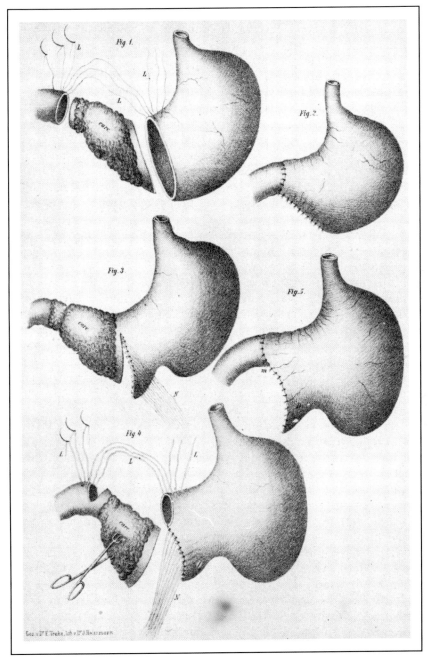

The stages of the gastrectomy on Frau Heller
From T. Billroth *Clinical Surgery. Extracts from the reports of Surgical Practice between the years 1860–1876.* London, the New Sydenham Society 1891

assistants were fully aware of the importance of our undertaking, and there was not the slightest disturbance, and not a minute of unnecessary conversation.

The tumour, lying immediately above and slightly to the right, seemed to be about as large as a medium-sized apple. Because of its size it was difficult to expose. It proved to be a partly nodular and partly infiltrated carcinoma of the pylorus and over a third of the lower part of the stomach. Adhesions with the omentum and transverse colon were divided. The small and large omentum were carefully separated. Every blood vessel was tied before it was divided. The loss of blood was extremely small. The entire tumour was moved on to the abdominal wall. Incision through the stomach 1 cm proximal to the infiltrated part, at first only at the back, then also through the duodenum. An attempt to bring the cut edges together showed that union was possible. Six sutures were passed through the edges of the wound. The threads were not yet tied, but only used to hold the edges of the wound in position. Further incision of the stomach, obliquely from above downwards and outwards, always 1 cm from the infiltrated part of the stomach. Now the oblique wound in the stomach was sutured from below upwards until the opening was only of a size that would fit the duodenum. Then the whole tumour was separated from the duodenum 1 cm beyond the infiltration by an incision parallel to that in the stomach (as in oval amputation). The duodenum was accurately inserted in the opening left in the stomach. About 50 stitches with Czerny carbolized silk. Cleansing with 2% carbolic acid solution. Revision of the whole suture. Auxillary stitches placed at points which seemed weak. Replacement in the abdominal cavity. Closure of the abdominal wound. Dressing.

Including the slowly administered anaesthesia the operation lasted 1½ hours. No weakness, no vomiting, no pain after the operation. For the first 24 hours nothing but ice was given by mouth. Then peptone enemas with wine. On the next day the patient was given a tablespoon of sour milk, at first every hour, then every half hour. The patient, a very sensible woman, feels quite well, lies unusually quietly, and sleeps most of the night with the help of a small injection of morphine. No wound pain; moderate febrile reaction. The dressing is still untouched. After some trials of broth, which the patient did not enjoy, feeding continues with sour milk only of which the patient takes about 1 litre a day. The enemas of peptone and pancreas easily cause flatulence and colic, and have therefore been stopped. A rectal injection of a little wine 2–3 times daily is agreeable to the patient. Yellowish, pulpy stools as in infants. The pulse is much quieter and fuller than before operation. This has continued up to now without the slightest complication. To prove how well she feels, I may add that I had to have her moved the day before yesterday to a large ward, at her own urgent request, because she found too little entertainment in the isolation ward which she shared with a woman, also bored, who had undergone ovariotomy on the same day.

The first resected specimen measures (horrible dictu!) 14 cm along the great curvature. The pylorus hardly admits a quill. The shape of the stomach is not much altered by the operation, but is merely smaller than before.

I am pleasantly astonished over the extremely smooth course; I expected more local and general reaction; I might almost say I expected more misbehaviour from the stomach. I still cannot quite believe that everything will continue so well. There could be a relapse into her prior debility—this would be the most fatal complication since nothing could be done about it. The wound and its surroundings must be by now, after six days, without reaction, nearly healed so that even if one or the other of the sutures should suppurate a general peritonitis would not be expected.

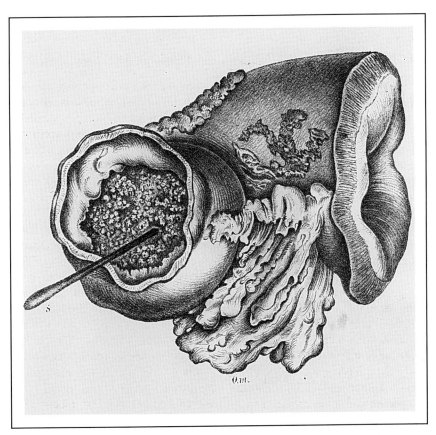

The resected specimen. A probe just passes through the malignant pyloric obstruction.

(From T. Billroth *Clinical Surgery. Extracts from the Reports of Surgical Practice between the years 1860–1876*. London, the New Sydenham Society 1891)

There could be local infection—abscesses around the scar. We hope that we shall discover them early enough so that we can drain them.

The course so far is already sufficient proof that the operation is possible. Our next care, and the subject of our next studies, must be to determine the indications, and to develop the technique to suit all kinds of cases. I hope we have taken another good step forward toward securing unfortunate people hitherto regarded as incurable, or, if there should be recurrences of cancer, at least alleviating their suffering for a time, and I am sure you will forgive me if I take solemn pride in the fact that it is the work of my pupils which has made this progress possible. *Nunquam retrosum* was the favourite motto of my teacher, Bernhard von Langenbeck, it must also be mine and my pupils.'

References

Billroth T. Open letter to Dr L. Wittelshöfer. *Wiener Medizinische Wochenschrift* 1881; **31**: 162.

Rutledge RH. In commemoration of Theodor Billroth on the 150th anniversary of his birth. *Surgery* 1979; **86**: 672–693.

Carl Langenbuch
The first cholecystectomy (1882)

In the present exciting climate of laparoscopic cholecystectomies, any surgeon with the slightest trace of interest in the historical roots of his craft must surely wish to read the case report of the first and extremely successful extirpation of the gall bladder. The date—July 15th 1882; the place—the Lazarus Hospital, Berlin; the surgeon—Carl Langenbuch.

Carl Johann Langenbuch was born in Kiel in 1846 and graduated from its university at the age of 23. His doctoral dissertation was on rupture of

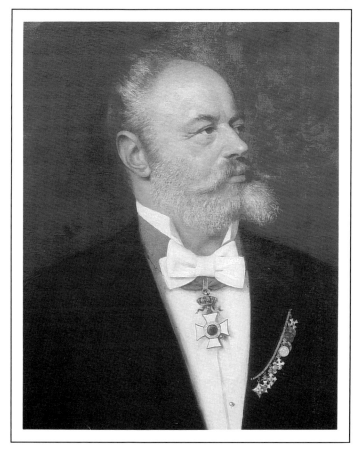

Carl Langenbuch
(Photograph provided by Dr Busso Maska, Lazarus Hospital, Berlin)

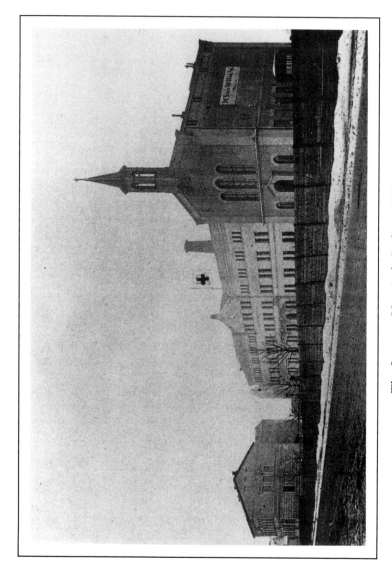

The Lazarus Hospital, Berlin, 1870

(Courtesy of Dr K. J. Hardy, Melbourne, Australia and the editor, *Australian and New Zealand Journal of Surgery*) the aorta. His surgical training was under Friedrich von Esmarch, (of tourniquet fame), at Kiel and under Wilms in Berlin. In 1873, at the age of only 27, he was appointed surgeon to the Lazarus Hospital. Langenbuch died in harness in 1901 of peritonitis due to appendicitis.

The operation of cholecystotomy for stones, first performed by John Bobbs in 1867 (see chapter 5) and popularised by Marion Sims, Theodor Kocher in Berne, WW Keen in Philadelphia and Lawson Tait in Birmingham, had the disadvantages of the problems of fistula formation, recurrent infection and residual stones.

Langenbuch believed the problem could be solved by extirpation of the organ and studied the procedure in a scientific manner in the autopsy room. He noted that elephants and horses do not possess this organ, and therefore concluded that man, too, could do without it! The operation he devised in his cadaver experiments was carried out through a T-shaped incision; the transverse limb was placed along the inferior margin of the liver and was joined to a longitudinal incision along the lateral margin of the rectus. The cystic duct was ligated with silk 1–2 cm from the gall bladder. The gall bladder was then dissected free from the liver bed, the bile emptied by aspiration to prevent spill and only then was the cystic duct transected.

Having carried out these preliminary *post mortem* studies, the time came for the living experiment. Herewith the case history:

C Langenbuch "A case of extirpation of the gallbladder for chronic cholecystitis. Cure"

Berlin Klinische Wochenschrift 1882; 19: 725–7

'At the end of June of this year my colleague, Dr N. Meyer, was kind enough to refer one of his patients to me for consultation—Mr D, 43 years old, Magistrate Secretary in Berlin, who suffered from severe gallstone symptoms. Never seriously ill before, in 1866 he was suddenly seized by persistent vomiting and severe colicky pain, which did not subside until the next day. At the beginning he had such attacks only 1–2 times a year. In 1869 severe jaundice, which subsided only after two months, appeared at the same time. From this point on the attacks of pain occurred more frequently and with greater intensity, were always followed by yellow colouring of the skin or at least of the conjunctiva and led to serious professional inconvenience. At one time a taut swelling in the gallbladder was thought palpable through the abdominal wall. Gallstones which were passed and found by chance were only a few dark-coloured specimens about the size of a pea. On the advice of Geh. Rath Frerichs, the patient visited Carlsbad for three consecutive years, but the pain increased rather than diminished. The first year the patient still weighed 89.5, a year ago only 75 and currently 54.2 kilos. There was thus considerable emaciation. The skin was flaccid and yellowish in colour, as was also the conjunctiva. There was a tendency to perspire. The tongue was not coated and the abdomen was soft. Liver dullness was within normal limits and the gallbladder area was not tender. The function of the extremely sensitive stomach was very subdued. The appetite was poor and there was a great tendency to vomiting and stubborn constipation. At the time neither bile components nor other abnormal impurities were detectable in the urine. Recently the attacks of pain recurred almost daily and often became so intense that they caused fainting spells on several occasions. For nine months the patient had treated these with increasing doses of morphine. In addition, he had become very depressed. He complained that his suffering had become increasingly worse, that he felt his strength diminishing and that he could no longer manage without morphine: he was considering giving up his job and was facing a bleak future.

The condition of the patient was in fact very precarious. The increasing weakness, the constant pain, the pronounced deterioration of the absorption of food and especially the increasing morphinism indicated that he was on a downward path from which return seemed almost impossible. Because the diagnosis was certain and the prognosis appeared so poor, I felt it was justified to make the patient aware of the one expedient which seemed possible to me and after presenting the pro and contra to him, to suggest that he think over further what he had heard.

After some time, during which he appears to have looked around still elsewhere for good advice, he was admitted (July 10th) to the Lazarus Hospital and requested that I perform the operation discussed. I had him stay in bed for five days and purged him in preparation. During this time he had two severe attacks daily, in which the pain clearly originated from the gallbladder area and then spread out over the abdomen.

The operation was arranged for July 15th. I need say no more about preparations for the ensuring of asepsis than that they were unusually careful in accordance with the newness of the procedure.

Besides my assistants and the necessary hospital personnel, my friends and colleagues Dr A. Martin, who kindly assisted and Dr F. Busch, as well as a few other guests were also present.

The operation proceeded exactly in the manner described above. The gallbladder did not appear to be affected by fresh inflammation but its walls were distinctly thickened. The gallbladder was only moderately filled with bile and was emptied by aspiration with a large Pravaz syringe. When opened, only two small cholesterol stones the size of a millet seed were found in it and it may be assumed that the several days' purging contributed to a thorough evacuation of stones. Upon separation of the gallbladder from the liver, insignificant venous bleeding occurred from the latter; it was easily stopped by a catgut suture.

The patient had no pain after the operation and slept well the following night.

On the morning of July 16th he was found with a lighted cigar in his mouth. At noon a strong feeling of hunger occurred, but only a minimum of light food was given. No pain the entire day. Temperature and pulse normal.

On July 17th a strong feeling of hunger occurred again, but as a precaution only a little liquid was given. No pain. Temperature and pulse normal.

On July 19th the patient feels a sharp pain under and between the shoulder blades during breathing. At 4.00 in the afternoon his temperature is 38.6 and his pulse 110. A thorough examination of the lungs is not done out of consideration of the abdominal wound: dry pleurisy is assumed. A warm water enema and a cup of St Germain tea are prescribed for constipation.

July 20th still no evacuation of the bowels, otherwise once again well being and normal temperature and pulse.

July 21st a few sutures are removed from the wound, which has already healed, and laxatives are again given. Towards evening very relieving liquid stools were passed.

Recovery progressed without interruption, so that the patient was already able to get out of bed on July 27th. As expected, the old pains have not recurred to date (middle of November) but, in contrast, the sensitive weakness of the stomach had to be treated for some time longer. However, even this subsided. Morphine has never been given again since the operation. By August 10th there had already been a weight gain of 6 kilos and a few weeks later upon discharge at the beginning of September a further gain of 7.5 kilos . . .

In the cases in question, even with only the minimum chance of danger to life now, cholecystectomy is preferable to resigning the patient to morphine and the incalculable turns of this insidious disease. In closing, if we yet review the cholecystotomies and cholelithectomies which were hitherto performed exclusively for the removal of hydrops, empyema and stones of the gallbladder, i.e. the opening of the gallbladder with subsequent suturing of the incised border to the abdominal wall, then it appears that these methods, by virtue of the opening of the abdominal cavity *mutatis mutandis,* are more dangerous than cholecystectomy because of the manipulation of the gallbladder! Because, on the one hand, there is the danger of leakage of secretion and possibly also of bile, as well as atmospheric air, into the abdominal cavity if the sutures give way; moreover, cholelithectomies can lead to protracted biliary fistulas with their disadvantages, and finally the disease will not be permanently cured in most cases because a recurrence of hydrops can occur if the mucous membrane has not been destroyed, and a new formation of stones can occur in the case of persistent patency of the cystic duct after occlusion of the gallbladder. I believe, therefore, that I may state that the extirpation of the gallbladder, performed by me for insidious cholelithiasis, after preceding litigation of the cystic duct, may be regarded as the less dangerous and more effective method, as well as for most other disease processes of this organ.'

References

Langenbuch CJA. A case of extirpation of the gallbladder for chronic cholecystitis. Cure. *Berlin Klinische Wochenschrift* 1882; **19**: 725–7.

Hardy KJ. Carl Langenbuch and the Lazarus Hospital: Events and circumstances surrounding the first cholecystectomy. *Australian and New Zealand Journal of Surgery* 1993; 63, 56–64.

Robinson JO. *Silvergirl's Surgery: Biliary Tract.* Austin: Silvergirl, 1985.

[10]

Sir William Arbuthnot Lane
Transabdominal cardiac massage (1902)

William Arbuthnot Lane was, with little doubt, one of the most colourful and controversial figures in British surgery. A brilliant surgeon, an innovator and a pioneer he was revered by his junior staff. He was also capable of setting up a violent antigen-antibody reaction with many of his peers.

Lane was born in 1846 at Fort St George, Scotland, where his father, an Army surgeon, was stationed at the time. He entered Guy's Hospital, London, at the early age of 16, qualified at the age of 21, and then was appointed house surgeon to the Victoria Hospital for Children in Chelsea. It was here he made his first contribution to operative surgery. He published five cases of rib resection for chronic empyema in children, with four successes. He returned to Guy's Hospital as demonstrator in anatomy in 1882 and stayed there for five years, laying down his intimate knowledge of anatomy that

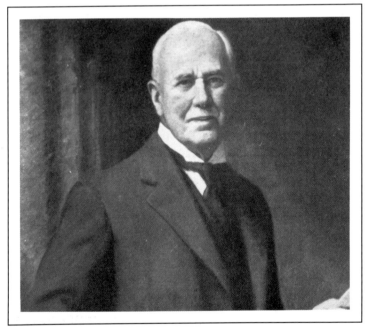

Sir William Arbuthnot Lane
(Reproduced by permission of the Principal, United Medical and Dental
Schools of Guy's and St Thomas's Hospitals)

flavoured much of his subsequent work. At the same time, he was appointed to the staff of the Hospital for Sick Children, Great Ormond Street. In 1888, he was elected to the consultant staff at Guy's Hospital and served it until his retirement in 1920.

Lane made important technical advances in many branches of surgery. He developed an ingenious operation for cleft palate, introduced antrectomy in the treatment of chronic purulent otitis media, and was first to treat septic thrombosis of the lateral cerebral sinus complicating mastoid infection by ligature of the internal jugular vein and removal of the septic thrombus. He was an early advocate of the use of saline for transfusion in the days before blood was available and, in 1909, he devised an operation for excision of a tumour of the cervical oesophagus, repairing the gap with local skin flaps.

Undoubtedly his greatest contribution was his pioneer work on the open fixation of fractures for which he devised his special perforated steel strips (Lane's plates). Any infection in such operations would, of course, prove disastrous, but Lane introduced the strictest asepsis into his operating theatre, the so-called 'no-touch technique', for which he devised special long artery and dissecting forceps so that, even in the deepest wound, the surgeon's fingers would not touch the wound edges. Although, in his day, Lane came in for powerful criticism for converting closed fractures into open wounds, his results spoke for themselves. Modern operative orthopaedic surgery owes much to his early efforts.

At the beginning of the twentieth century, Lane became obsessed with the concept that chronic constipation ('intestinal stasis') produced toxaemia and that this 'auto-intoxication' was the cause of most of the ills of civilized mankind. Lane claimed that stasis, largely by facilitating infection of the upper alimentary canal, resulted in duodenal ulcer, pancreatitis, alimentary cancer and gallstones, as well as degenerative disease of the heart, blood vessels and kidneys, mental disturbances, rheumatoid arthritis, and, indeed a whole catalogue of other syndromes. He first carried out a complete short-circuit of the large intestine by means of an ileorectal anastomosis. He then went even further and carried out total colectomy in patients with conditions ranging from migraine to rheumatism. Not unnaturally, his views were violently opposed by many of his colleagues.

Fortunately, as the years passed, Lane decided that patients could keep the colon as long as it was kept empty. He then introduced liquid paraffin into the pharmacopoea. At least this was safer for the patient than a total colectomy!

Eventually, Lane removed his name from the Medical Register so that he could address the public by lectures and through the press on his ideas for health. He founded the New Health Society whose aims were to teach the public the simple laws of health, to attempt to make fruit and vegetables inexpensive and abundant, and to encourage people to go back to the land. He might be regarded as a pioneer of what is now called 'social medicine'.

Lane went on lecturing until the outbreak of World War II. He died in 1943 at the ripe old age of 86.

Among Lane's achievements was a 'first' that seems hardly to have registered with him as particularly important because he never actually published the case. This was the first successful resuscitation by cardiac massage.

Moritz Schiff in 1874 first demonstrated that dogs, in which cardiac arrest had been induced by chloroform, could be resuscitated by rhythmic compression of the exposed heart. By 1901, a dozen attempts had been reported of open cardiac massage in man without success. Lane's successful case of transabdominal transdiaphragmatic massage appeared in a report of the proceedings of the Society of Anaesthetists in the *Lancet* of 1902:

Leading Article "Resuscitation in syncope due to anaesthetics and in other conditions by rhythmical compression of the heart"

Lancet 1902; 2: 1476

'At the last meeting of the Society of Anaesthetists, Dr E. A. Starling reported the case of a man aged 65 years, whose appendix vermiformis was removed under nitrous oxide and ether. During the trimming of the stump both pulse and respiration stopped together. Artificial respiration and traction on the tongue were performed without success. Then the surgeon, Mr W. Arbuthnot Lane, introduced his hand through the abdominal incision and felt the motionless heart through the diaphragm. He gave it a squeeze or two and felt it re-start beating, though no radial pulse was discernable. As voluntary respiration was still suspended, artificial respiration was continued and other restorative measures were adopted. Artificial respiration had to be continued for about 12 minutes when natural respiration recommenced with a long-sighing respiration, while at the same time the pulse became perceptible. The operation was completed without any more anaesthetic and good convalescence followed though there was some diaphragmatic tenderness. It should be noted that the method adopted by Dr Starling, whom we congratulate, differs from those previously employed. Instead of incising the diaphragm as recommended by Mauclaire he adopted the simpler method of compressing the heart through the diaphragm. The previous results of manual compression of the heart are not very encouraging, but Mr. Lane's success by such a simple and easy procedure justifies us in saying that if at laparotomy a patient's heart stops the case should never be abandoned as hopeless until manual compression of the heart through the diaphragm has been performed.'

References

Ellis H. *Notable Names in Medicine and Surgery*. 4th Edition. London: Lewis, 1983
Layton TB. *Sir William Arbuthnot Lane*. Edinburgh: Livingstone, 1956.
Leading Article. Resuscitation in syncope due to anaesthetics and in other conditions by rhythmical compression of the heart. *Lancet* 1902; ii: 1476

[11]
Sir Henry Sessions Souttar
The first transauricular mitral valvotomy (1925)

Even cardiac surgeons might not know that the first, and entirely successful, transauricular mitral valvotomy was performed as long ago as 1925. The surgeon was Henry Souttar, a general surgeon who operated without the advantages of antibiotic cover, blood transfusion or sophisticated anaesthetic equipment.

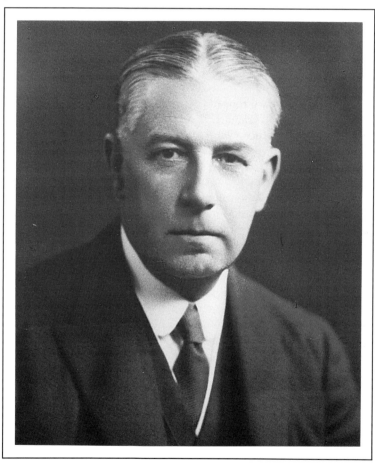

Sir Henry Sessions Souttar
(Reproduced by permission of the President and Council of the Royal College of Surgeons of England)

The patient, a girl of 15, a labourer's daughter, under the care of Lord Dawson, made an uneventful recovery and lived in very fair health for five years. She then had a cerebral infarct, probably from a clot in the left auricular appendage, from which she died.

The medical establishment was solidly against such an intervention—no matter how successful—and Souttar never got another case!

Henry Souttar was born in 1875, the son of a Scottish member of Parliament. He studied mathematics and engineering at the University of Oxford, where he obtained a double first. He became a clinical student at the London Hospital Medical School and qualified in 1906, taking his final FRCS three years later. He then demonstrated in Anatomy at his medical school, became surgical registrar at the London and was appointed to the staff of the West London Hospital in 1912. Three years later he was appointed to the staff of the London Hospital.

On the outbreak of World War I he went to Belgium as Surgeon-in-Chief to a Field Hospital and carried out excellent surgical work at the siege of Antwerp. Fortunately, he was able to escape with his field ambulance and spent the rest of the war as a surgeon in the RAMC in England.

His mathematical knowledge and engineering skill, together probably with the influence of his father-in-law, who was Professor of Physics at Oxford, were no doubt responsible for his skill in devising many surgical instruments and for his interest in radium. Perhaps best known is his technique for intubation of oesophageal tumours, for which he devised and made in his own workshop his ingenious metal wire tube. This, of course, was the forerunner of modern palliative intubation. When radium was first discovered he went to Paris to meet the Curies and wrote much on this subject. He devised a special introducer for the insertion of radon seeds.

Souttar's later career remained distinguished. He served on the Council of the Royal College of Surgeons from 1933–1949 and during the Second World War was Chairman of the Central Medical War Committee. In 1945 he became President of the British Medical Association. He was knighted in 1949. Souttar died in 1964 aged nearly 89. He had passed his time in his seventies by constructing for himself a planetarium. His place in history, however, must be the operation he performed on the 16th May 1925. It was to be 22 years before this operation, of mitral valvotomy, was to be repeated.

HS Souttar "The surgical treatment of mitral stenosis"

British Medical Journal 1925; 2: 603–6

'There can be no more fascinating problem in surgery than the relief of pathological conditions of the valves of the heart. Despite the consecutive changes to which these lesions may have given rise in the cardiac muscle, the relief of the lesions themselves would undoubtedly be of immense service to the patient and must be followed by marked improvement in his general condition. Expressed in these terms, the problem is to a large extent mechanical, and as such should already be within the scope of surgery, were it not for the extraordinary nature of the conditions under which the problem must be attacked. We are, however, of the opinion that these conditions again are purely mechanical, and that apart from them the heart is as amenable to surgical treatment as any other organ. Incisions can be made into its chambers, portions of its structure can be excised, and internal manipulations can be carried out, without the slightest interference with its action, and there is ample evidence that wounds of the heart heal as rapidly as those in any other region.

The conditions which appear as fundamental are, first, that the operations have to be carried out on a structure in rapid movement; and secondly, that no interference whatever with the circulation must take place. The first is not quite so difficult as it sounds, for it is possible to fix the actual portion of the heart which is under operation, but it must obviously limit the possibilities of repair. In animals the second condition may sometimes be ignored, and the circulation has been clamped for as much as two minutes. This, however, would never be justifiable in a human being, in view of the extreme danger to the brain from even the shortest check to its blood supply. Any manipulations which are carried out must therefore be executed in the full flow of the blood stream, and they must not perceptibly interfere with the contractions of the heart.

The simplest valvular lesion for surgical interference is stenosis of one of the valves, and of these the mitral valve is perhaps the most accessible. I have been interested for some time in the development of a suitable technique for reaching this valve, and I owe to Dr Otto Leyton the opportunity presented by the following case for putting my ideas to the test. A description of the case itself will give the clearest indication of the method of approach I adopted and of the technique which I devised.

Description of Case

L.H., aged 15, was admitted to the London Hospital in January, 1921, suffering from chorea and mitral stenosis. Her subsequent history was one of many relapses, with steadily increasing failure of compensation. In September, 1924, she was admitted with haemoptysis, vomiting and severe dyspnoea. She was cyanosed, her feet were swollen, and her liver was enlarged and tender. After three weeks in hospital she had greatly improved and was sent to a convalescent home, whence three weeks later she was discharged.

Early in March 1925, she appeared at the London Hospital with cough, dyspnoea, and pain in the limbs. She went home to bed and given digitalis and aspirin, but she did not improve. After a severe attack of epistaxis and precordial pain she was again admitted as an in-patient.

She was a thin girl with a bright malar flush. Her pulse rate was 128, and respirations 32. Cardiac pulsation was visible over a large area of the left chest, and the rib cartilages in this area were very soft and had a forward bulge. The apex beat was in the fifth space, outside the mid-clavicular line, and the area of cardiac dullness extended to the second space above. In the mitral area there was a long rumbling diastolic murmur, followed by a soft blowing systolic murmur, the latter being conducted out into the axilla. A presystolic murmur was present, but was not very marked. The liver was not obviously enlarged, but was slightly tender on palpation.

After a week's rest in bed her pulse fell to 80 and her respirations to 24, while her general condition greatly improved. Her pulse was now small but perfectly regular with a systolic pressure of 95mm. There was no presystolic murmur or thrill, but a long diastolic murmur of low pitch was followed by a soft blowing systolic murmur.

In view of her many relapses it appeared that her heart was unable to establish compensation for the combined stenosis and regurgitation from which she suffered, and it was therefore decided to attempt to relieve the stenosis by surgical means.

Operation.

On May 6th, 1925, under intratracheal anaesthesia, a curved incision was made along the fourth left intercostal space, up along the middle of the sternum, and outwards along the first intercostal space. The skin and subcutaneous tissues, with the left breast, were turned outwards, exposing an area of the chest wall about five inches square. On the outer side of this area a short horizontal incision was made along each of the three ribs exposed (Fig 1), and through these incisions the ribs were in turn divided. The chest wall was now divided a little within the line of the original incision by cutting through the muscles and costal cartilages, and the flap so formed was turned outwards, the pleura being included in the flap (Fig 2).

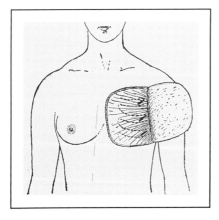

Figure 1

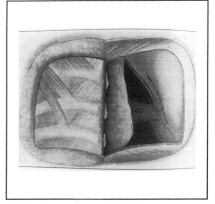

Figure 2

A very full exposure of the left pericardium was thus obtained, while with an intratracheal pressure of 15 mmHg there was only moderate collapse of the left lung. The action of the heart now became extremely hurried, the pulse rising to 150 and it was evident that until it settled down nothing further could be attempted. After five minutes' delay the beats became slower and steadier, and it was decided that we could safely proceed. The pericardium was opened by a vertical incision three inches long, in the centre of which the left auricular appendage came prominently forward (Fig 3). Two sutures were passed through the upper and lower margins of the appendage, so that it could be readily drawn forward. As the heart was still beating very rapidly the wound was covered with hot saline pads and a subcutaneous injection of 1/100 grain of strophanthin was given. After a delay of ten minutes the heart had steadied down to a rate of 120, and the blood pressure, which had fallen to 60mm, had returned to 90mm.

The auricular appendage was now drawn forward, a soft curved clamp (Fig 4) was applied to its base, and it was incised in an antero-posterior

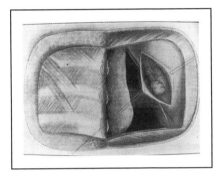

Figure 3

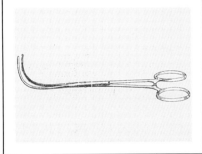

Figure 4

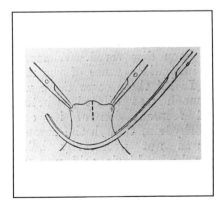

Figure 5

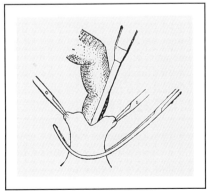

Figure 6

direction with scissors (Fig 5). Into this opening the left forefinger was inserted (Fig 6), the clamp was withdrawn, and the appendage was drawn over the finger like a glove by means of the sutures. The whole of the inside of the left auricle could now be explored with facility. It was immediately evident from the rush of blood against the finger that gross regurgitation was taking place, but there was not so much thickening of the valves as had been expected. The finger was passed into the ventricle through the orifice of the mitral valve without encountering resistance, and the cusps of the valve could be easily felt and their condition estimated.

The finger was kept in the auricle for perhaps two minutes, and during that time, so long as it remained in the auricle, it appeared to produce no effect upon the heart beat of the pulse. The moment, however, that it passed into the orifice of the mitral valve the blood pressure fell to zero, although even then no change in the cardiac rhythm could be detected. The blood stream was simply cut off by the finger, which presumably just fitted the stenosed orifice. As, however, the stenosis was of such moderate degree, and was accompanied by so little thickening of the valves, it was decided not to carry out the valve section which had been arranged, but to limit intervention to such dilation as could be carried out by the finger. It was felt that an actual section of the valve might only make matters worse by increasing the degree of regurgitation, while the breaking down of adhesions by the finger might improve the condition as regards both regurgitation and stenosis.

It was now decided to withdraw the finger and close the appendage. Unfortunately, at the critical moment of withdrawal the lower retaining suture cut through, the appendage slipped back into the pericardium, and there was a sudden gush of blood, which, however, was instantly checked by pressing the appendage against the heart. With a little manipulation the tip of the appendage was now grasped between the finger and the thumb, which held it securely closed while an assistant passed a silk ligature round it and tied it off. The pericardium was closed, and a certain amount of blood, which in this contretemps had escaped into the pleural cavity, was removed with moist gauze pads. The wound was closed in layers, the ribs being accurately sutured in position. Before the flap was actually closed a small quantity of 60 per cent alcohol was injected into the intercostal nerves just outside the point at which the ribs had been divided.

Immediately the chest was closed the heart's action returned to normal, and on the conclusion of the operation the general condition of the patient was indistinguishable from that at the beginning. She had a bright colour and an excellent pulse. Except at the moment when the suture cut out, her condition had never caused the slightest anxiety, and even then there was only a momentary drop in the blood pressure. The whole operation took precisely sixty minutes.

She made an uninterrupted recovery, the freedom from pain or any disturbance which might have been expected to result from the operation being remarkable. Her general condition appeared to be greatly improved, but the physical signs showed little or no change. She was sent to the country and kept in bed for six weeks, but as at the end of that time her pulse rate remained constant at about 90 she was gradually allowed to get up. At the end of three months, she declared that she felt perfectly well, although she still became somewhat breathless on exertion.

Remarks

I believe that this is the first occasion upon which an attempt has been made to reach the mitral valve by this route in the human being, or to subject the interior of the heart to digital examination. The value of the method cannot possibly be judged on a single case, but I think that I may claim to have shown that the method is practicable and that it is reasonably safe. Indeed, the features which most struck all who were present at the operation were the facility and the absolute safety of the whole procedure, while even on a first attempt the amount and precision of the information to be gained by digital

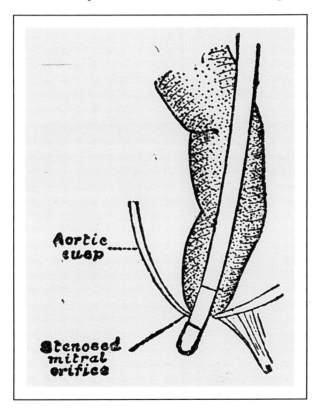

Figure 7
(Figures 1–7 reproduced by permission of the *British Medical Journal*)

exploration were very remarkable. I had intended to divide the aortic cusp by passing a thin hernia bistoury along my finger (Fig 7) and thus to relieve the stenosis, and this could have been done with perfect facility had it been considered advisable.

The problem of cardiac surgery had frequently attracted the attention of both physicians and surgeons, and two years ago the *British Medical Journal* summed up, in an admirable article, its history and position at that time. It is now being attacked with characteristic energy by several American surgeons from various points of view. On the experimental side Duff Allen, by means of a most ingenious optical device, has succeeded in actually seeing the mitral valve in the cat and in dividing a cusp, using the approach through the auricular appendage. On the clinical side, Cutler, after an elaborate experimental investigation, succeeded in excising portions of stenosed mitral valves in human beings by means of an ingenious valvulotome, working through the ventricle. The operation was, however, necessarily blind and proved to be somewhat dangerous.

It appears to me that the method of digital exploration through the auricular appendage cannot be surpassed for simplicity and directness. Not only is the mitral orifice directly to hand, but the aortic valve itself is most certainly within reach, through the mitral orifice. Owing to the simplicity of the structures, and oddly enough, to their constant and regular movement, the information given by the finger is exceedingly clear, and personally I felt an appreciation of the mechanical reality of stenosis and regurgitation which I never before possessed. To hear a murmur is a very different matter from feeling the blood itself pouring back over one's finger. I could not help being impressed by the mechanical nature of these lesions and by the practicability of their surgical relief.'

References

Hurwitz A, Degenshein GA. *Milestones in Modern Surgery.* Sir Henry Souttar— Biographical Sketch. p 409. New York: Hoeber and Harper, 1958.

Robinson RHOB, Le Fanu WR. *Lives of the Fellows of the Royal College of Surgeons of England 1952–1964.* Sir Henry Sessions Souttar. p 390–2. Edinburgh: Livingstone, 1970.

Souttar HS. The surgical treatment of mitral stenosis. *British Medical Journal* 1925; 2: 603–606.

[12]

Charles Dubost

Resection of an aortic aneurysm (1951)

On 11th January 1991 a great surgical pioneer, Charles Dubost, died at the age of 76. Forty years previously he performed the first successful resection of an abdominal aortic aneurysm. This report greatly influenced general and vascular surgeons throughout the world who, until then, had regarded this entity as being outside the bounds of surgical removal and reconstruction. Indeed, as a young surgeon myself, I could hardly believe such an operation possible, having seen primitive attempts at dealing with this formidable problem by introducing coils of wire into the aneurysmal sac or otherwise having stood by and watched the patient exsanguinate from his ruptured anuerysm.

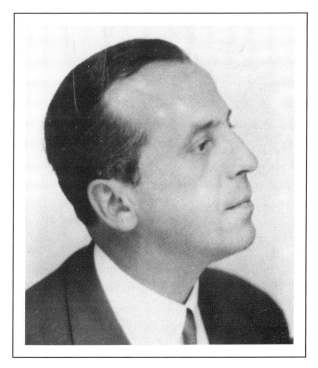

Charles Dubost
(From P. Blondeau Necrologie de Charles Dubost. *La Presse Médicale* 1991; **20**: 397–8. Paris: Masson, with permission of the publishers)

Charles Dubost was born in 1914 in the Latin Quarter of Paris, where his father was a pharmacist. He studied in the capital city, won the Croix de Guerre as a young medical lieutenant in the early days of World War II and then joined the Hôpital Broussais after the war as a general surgeon. In 1947 he commenced cardiac surgery in a small special 'blue baby' unit at this hospital.

His classical paper on aneurysm was first presented on September 18th 1951 in La Semaine des Hôpitaux de Paris and was reprinted in translation in *Archives of Surgery* in 1952.

Dubost was internationally recognized as a leading cardiac surgeon of France. He became an officer of la Legion d'honneur and was elected both to the Academy of Medicine and Academy of Science.

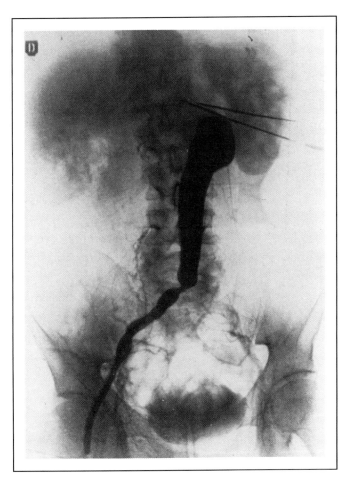

The pre-operative aortogram
(Reproduced by permission of La Semaine des Hôpitaux)

Charles Dubost, Michel Allary and Nicolas Oeconomos
"Resection of an aneurysm of the abdominal aorta reestablishment of the continuity by a preserved human arterial graft, with result after five months"

Archives of Surgery 1952; 64: 405–8

'Mr Le G, aged 50 years, had an aneurysm of the abdominal aorta revealed by gross disturbances of function, predominantly in the left leg. Abdominal examination showed a large tumour in the left paraumbilical region, pulsating and expansile. The right femoral pulse was diminished and the left absent; oscillations were diminished on the right and absent on the left. One year before he had a myocardial infarction. The blood Wassermann test was negative. The aortograph shows that the beginning of the aneurysm is just below the kidneys and that it extends as far as the bifurcation of the aorta. The left common iliac artery is blocked in its first 5 or 6 cm. The right common iliac artery, although patent, has as its origin two small aneurysmal dilatations. The superior mesenteric and renal arteries, perfectly delineated by the opaque medium, are clearly above the aneurysm. The inferior mesenteric artery, however, is not injected.

Operative Intervention (March 29, 1951, Dr Dubost)—A left thoracoabdominal incision was made, an extra peritoneal approach being used, and resection of the 11th rib was carried out. Retraction of the peritoneal sac disclosed an enormous aneurysm extending from the origin

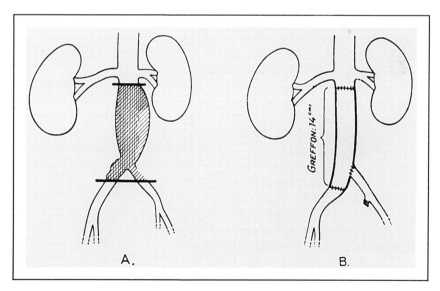

The operative drawings
(Reproduced by permission of La Semaine des Hôpitaux)

of the renal arteries to the common iliac arteries. It was decided to attempt its complete removal and to use a graft to reestablish continuity of the arteries.

The operation was carried out in the following stages: Control of the aneurysm was obtained by a clamp proximally to it, immediately below the renal arteries. Next, in the region of the iliac arteries, came exposure, isolation, and provisional haemostasis of both external iliac and both internal iliac arteries. Section of both common iliac arteries was performed and then dissection of the aneurysm from below upward. The stripping was troublesome near the common iliac veins and the inferior vena cava, which were adherent in places to the aneurysmal sac, fragments of which had to be left in some places. The lumbar vessels, thrombosed, were sectioned without ligature. The inferior mesenteric artery did not bleed from the proximal cut end but did spout blood from the peripheral end. The aneurysm, entirely freed, was turned upward and sectioned 2 cm from the clamp on the aorta.

The cut end of the aorta proximally and the cut end of the right common iliac artery peripherally were trimmed in order to interpose the graft (15 cm in length and taken from the thoracic aorta of a 20 year old girl three weeks previously). The superior anastomosis of the aortic graft was carried out with 5/0 silk.

Since we did not have a Y-shaped graft, it was necessary to make an end-to-end anastomosis between the graft and the right common iliac artery.

The obstruction in the left common iliac artery was removed, and after section of the internal iliac artery, which was itself blocked, it was anastomosed to the side of the graft immediately above the other anastomosis. After removal of the clamps, the three anastomoses were widely patent, and the femoral pulses were felt to be equal on the two sides.

A check aortograph was carried out two months later and showed perfect function of the graft, which was not at all dilated but was widely patent, as were also the iliac and femoral arteries.

Three months after the operation the patient was in perfect health. The femoral pulses were strong and equal and also the posterior tibial and dorsalis pedis arteries. The specimen, 15 cm long was made up of a large sac with a very thin wall which was calcified in many places and was completely filled by a large clot which had a canal through its centre about 3 cm in diameter.

Histological Examination—The aortic wall, extremely altered, shows the following changes from the cavity of the aneurysm outward: There is a much thickened intima, transformed into an amorphous mass not taking up the stain, studded with fatty acid crystals, and showing calcareous degeneration in the deepest part. Immediately under the calcified areas is the beginning of the media, still recognizable in this region from several areas of elastic fibres which are fragmented. The outer four-fifths of the media are totally lacking in elastic tissue. In contrast, the muscle fibres are almost normal in appearance but fibrous tissue is more prominent. The main feature, together with the destruction of elastic tissue, is the presence throughout the outer half of the aorta of masses of lymphocytic cells accompanying the vasa vasorum; these cells form concentric sheets but also are seen sometimes to follow the vessels at right angles to the layers of the wall. This periarteritis is accompanied in places with endoarteritis obliterans, several vasa vasorum being completely obstructed.

No inflammatory sclerosis was seen.

In summary, the lesion is an aneurysm with marked changes in the walls and calcium deposition. The endarteritis and periarteritis of the vasa vasorum would suggest an inflammatory process without any specific indication as to its nature.

Conclusions

A case of aneurysm of the abdominal aorta extending from the renal to the iliac arteries is reported. The method chosen for its excision was a combined abdominothoracic approach on the left; this gave the necessary exposure of the aortic bifurcation and the origin of the renal arteries.

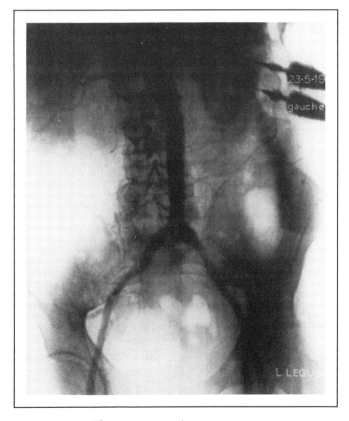

The post-operative aortogram
(Reproduced by permission of La Semaine des Hôpitaux)

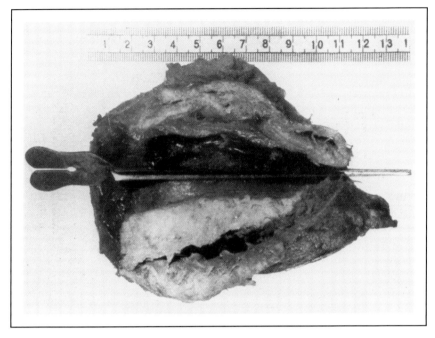

The resected specimen
(Reproduced by permission of La Semaine des Hôpitaux)

The reestablishment of continuity of the aorta was assured by a graft of human aorta which had been preserved for three weeks. An aortograph carried out two months after the operation showed perfect permeability of the graft as well as of the iliac arteries, of which the left one had been obstructed. Five months after surgical intervention the pulse and oscillations in both legs were normal and equal.'

References

Blondeau P. Nécrologie; Charles Dubost. *La Presse Médicale* 1991; **20**: 397–8.
Dubost C, Allary M, Oeconomos N. Resection of an aneurysm of the abdominal aorta. Reestablishment of the continuity by a preserved human arterial graft with result after five months. *Archives of Surgery* 1952; **64**: 405–8.

Part II
The Surgeon at War

[13]
Ambroise Paré
Treatment of gunshot wounds (1537)

Every time a military surgeon deals with a traumatized limb, he should utter a silent prayer to a 16th century French surgeon, Ambroise Paré. Among his many contributions, Paré did two great services for surgery and therefore for suffering mankind; first, he showed that gunshot wounds need not be

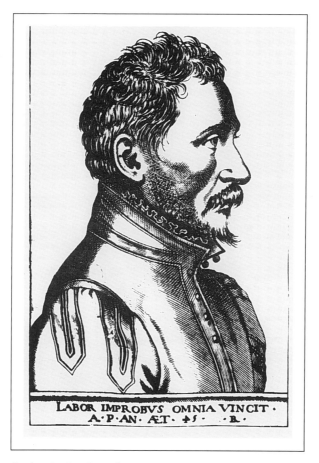

LABOR IMPROBVS OMNIA VINCIT·
A·P·AN· ÆT· 4*5* · ·B·

Ambroise Paré aged 45. Engraving attributed to Jean
Le Royer 1561
(Reproduced with permission of the Librarian, University
of Glasgow Library)

cauterized with boiling oil, and second, he replaced the red-hot iron with the ligature in the control of haemorrhage from great vessels during amputation. By these advances, both of which were based on close clinical observation and immense experience, he saved untold numbers of wounded soldiers from the tortures which had previously been inflicted upon them.

Paré was born in the little town of Laval in the Province of Maine in 1510. His father was probably *valet de chambre* and barber to the local squire and he may thus have obtained some interest in the work of the barber-surgeons. Paré's sister married a barber-surgeon who practised in Paris and his elder brother Jean was a master barber-surgeon in Vitré.

Ambroise may have begun the study of surgery with his brother and it is certain that he did work with a barber-surgeon in the provinces before coming to Paris at the age of 22 as an apprentice to a barber-surgeon. He soon was appointed *compagnon-chirurgeon*, roughly equivalent to house surgeon today, at the Hôtel-Dieu, which was then the only public hospital

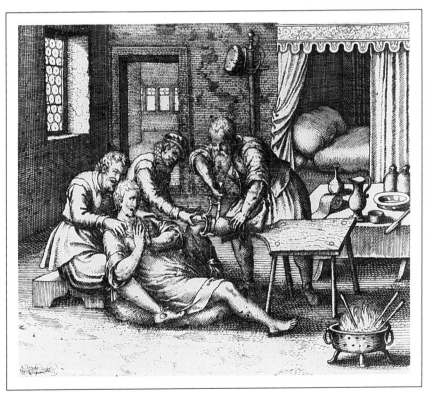

An amputation of the leg, 16th century. Note the cauteries heating in the brazier. It was Paré who replaced the cautery with the ligature
(*Degangreno et Sphacelo libre* Fabry von Hilden. Reproduced by permission of the President and Council, Royal College of Surgeons of England)

in Paris, where he worked for the next three or four years and must have gained great experience in that repository of pathology.

Perhaps because he could not afford to pay the fees for admission to the ranks of the barber-surgeons, Paré started his career at the age of 26 as a military surgeon. In those days, there was no organized medical care for the humble private soldiers of armies in the field. Surgeons were attached to individual generals and other important personages, and might, if they wished, give what aid they could to the common soldiers in their spare time.

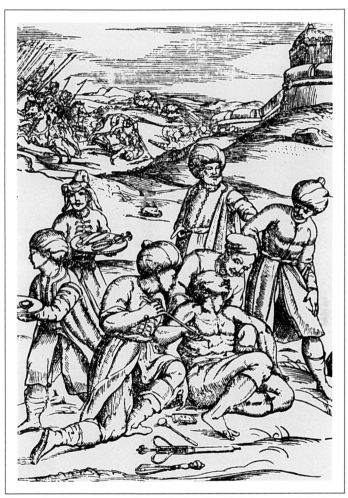

Cauterization of wounds on the battlefield. Giovanni Andrea della Croce *Chiruggiae universalis opus* Venice. R. Meiettus 1595
(Wellcome Institute Library, reproduced with permission of the Wellcome Institute, London)

Otherwise the troops had to rely on the rough and ready help of their companions or of a motley crowd of horse doctors, farriers, quacks, mountebanks and camp followers.

Paré was appointed surgeon to the Mareschal de Montejan, who was colonel-general of the French infantry. This, his first of many campaigns, took him to Turin, and it was here in 1537, that he made his fundamental observations on the treatment of gunshot wounds. He soon realized that the accepted method of treating these injuries with boiling oil did more harm than good and substituted a more humane and less destructive dressing.

Returning from his first campaign, Paré passed his examinations for admission to the Community of Barber-Surgeons in 1541, married and settled down in a practice in Paris. However, he was frequently called away into military service and, in all, was involved in 17 campaigns.

Ligation of major blood vessels was known to the ancients. Paré's only claim, as he makes quite clear in his own writings, was that he first applied this method in performing amputations, thereby ending the torture of the practice of cauterizing the stump with the red hot iron. Paré first employed the ligature in amputation of the leg in 1552 at the Siege of Danvillier.

Paré was surgeon to no less than four kings of France. He died in Paris in 1590 at the great age of 80. He remained throughout his life a simple, humble man. In his very first campaign he ended his description of the treatment of a gunshot wound of the ankle with perhaps his most famous phrase, 'I dressed the wound and God healed him'.

Paré was a prolific writer. He broke convention by writing in French and not in Latin, since indeed he had no knowledge of the latter. His best known work is his *Apologie and Treatise Containing the Voyages Made into Divers Places*, which was published in 1585 and amounts to an autobiography of his 50 years of military experiences.

It was in the *Apologie* that Paré describes the observations he made in the Turin campaign of 1537. It amounted to what today might well be described as one of the earliest controlled surgical experiments. How many of us have carried some new and untried treatment and have had this experience of being unable to sleep and have come into the ward before anyone else is around, with pulse racing, to see whether the treatment we have carried out has been a brilliant success or a disastrous failure.

Ambroise Paré, Geoffrey Keynes (Editor) "The apologie and treatise of Ambroise Paré containing the voyages made into divers places with many of his writings upon surgery"

London: Falcon Educational Books, 1951

'I was at that time a fresh-water surgeon, since I had not yet seen treated wounds made by firearms. It is true I had read in Jean deVigo in his first book of *Wounds in General* chapter 8, that wounds made by firearms are poisoned because of the powder. For their cure he advised their cauterization with oil of elders mixed with a little theriac. To not fail, this oil must be applied boiling, even though this would cause the wounded extreme pain. I wished to know first how to apply it, how the other surgeons did their first dressings, which was to apply the oil as boiling as possible. So I took heart to do as they did. Finally, my oil was exhausted and I was forced instead to apply a digestive made of egg yolk, rose oil and turpentine. That night I could not sleep easily, thinking that by failure of cauterizing, I would find the wounded in whom I had failed to put the oil dead of poisoning. This made me get up early in the morning to visit them. There, beyond my hope, I found those on whom I had used the digestive medication feeling little pain in their wounds, without inflammation and swelling, having rested well through the night. The others on whom I had used the oil I found feverish, with great pain, swelling and inflammation around their wounds. Then I resolved never again to so cruelly burn the poor wounded by gunshot.'

References

Ellis H. *Famous Operations*. Media, Pennsylvania: Harwal Publishing, 1984.
Keynes G. (Editor). *The Apologie and Treatise of Ambroise Paré containing the Voyages made into Divers Places with many of his writings upon Surgery.* London: Falcon Educational Books, 1951.

[14]
Richard Wiseman
Wounds of the brain (1686)

Every surgeon realizes that war injuries are particularly horrible. It is bad enough for people to be injured accidentally, but this is especially compounded when maiming follows man's inhumanity to man. We regard the trauma produced by modern instruments of war with particular dread—the high explosive shell, the rocket, the nerve gas, the chemical burn—but

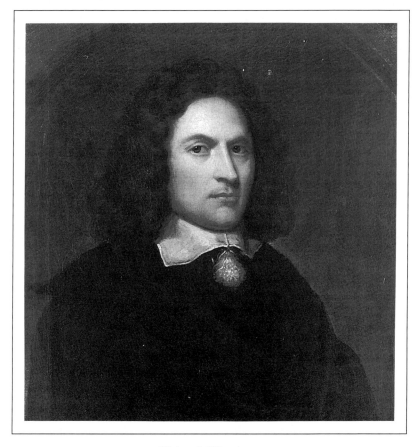

Richard Wiseman
(Reproduced by permission of the President and Council of the Royal College
of Surgeons of England)

the wounded of yester-year had no morphia instantly to assuage the pain, no helicopters for rapid rescue and no anaesthetics to mitigate the agony of the surgeon's knife.

The vivid case reports of Richard Wiseman bring this lesson home to us as well as any wartime writings of the past.

Wiseman was a colourful character whose life reads more like a novel than the biography of a distinguished surgeon. We do not even know the exact date or place of his birth and nothing of his parentage. We believe that he was born between 1621 and 1623 in or near London. The fact that nothing is known of his family indicates that he was probably illegitimate. He might well have been the bastard son of one or other of the Sir Richard Wisemans living in the Home Counties at that time who were of an age at which they could have fathered the future surgeon.

Certainly in 1637, Richard was apprenticed to Richard Smith, a surgeon, and following this he may have served in the Dutch Navy, although there are no certain facts to support this. In 1645, at the beginning of the Civil War between the Roundheads of Oliver Cromwell and the Cavaliers of Charles I, Wiseman was appointed surgeon to a Royalist battalion commanded by Colonel Ballard, which was raised in the South West of the country and he was present at the Battles of Taunton and Truro. With the defeat of these troops, Wiseman escaped and worked as a surgeon in exile in France and the Low Countries.

1649 saw the trial and execution by decapitation of Charles I. The following year his son, now Charles II, left Holland and landed with his followers in Scotland. He was accompanied by Richard Wiseman, who acted as surgeon at several bloody battles, including the Battle of Dunbar. At first, the troops of Charles II were victorious over Cromwell's Republican army and advanced into the Midlands of England but they were defeated in 1651 at the Battle of Worcester. Charles, after many adventures, managed to escape to the continent but many of his followers, including Wiseman, were captured and Richard spent many months in prison at Chester.

On his release from captivity, Wiseman was enrolled as Freeman of the Company of Barber Surgeons in London in 1652, where he practised as a civilian surgeon. However, he was imprisoned once again for some months and in 1654, on his release, his practice now ruined, he left for Spain and served in the Spanish Navy in the West Indies.

In 1660, Charles II returned to England and was restored to the throne. Within ten days of the King's entry into London, Wiseman was appointed his Surgeon in Ordinary. Five years later, he was appointed Master of the Company of Barber Surgeons and in 1672 he was appointed Sergeant Surgeon to the King.

In May 1676, Wiseman published his major work, by which he is remembered to this day, his *Several Chirurgical Treatises*, dedicated to Charles II. By now he was a very sick man and he died on 20th August of that year, probably from pulmonary tuberculosis.

Wiseman's vivid reports of front-line surgery are illustrated by these case notes in his section on Wounds of the Brain:

Richard Wiseman "Several chirurgical treatises"

Second Edition 1686, Book 5, Page 400

'At Sterling . . . a poor servant-maid came to me to be dressed of a wound she had received on her head by a musket shot in the taking of Calender-House by the enemy. There was a fracture with a depression of the skull. I set on a trepan for the elevation of the depressed bone, and for discharge of the sanies. She had laboured under this fracture at least a week before she came to me . . . after perforation, and raising up this depressed bone and dressing her wound, she went her way, and came daily thither to be dressed, as if it had been only a simple wound of the hairy scalp. Mr Penycuke, an eminent chirurgeon of that Nation, did assist me in this work. I think the brain itself was wounded. I left her in his hands, who I suppose finished the cure. At the beating up of our out-guards near Truro, the enemy pursuing them, a trooper wounded between right brow and ear, espying me amongst the crowd, importuned me earnestly to dress him, and would admit of no excuse. We stopped at an Apothecarie's House on the right hand going out of the town towards Perin. I called to the Apothecarie's servant to bring somewhat to dress him. Meanwhile I hastily lifed up the bloody hair, and saw a quantity of the brain lie among it. I took it up with my fingers, and showed it to him; the sight whereof so calmed his passion, that I had liberty to fly from the enemy who was entered the town.

At the siege of Melcomb-Regis, a foot soldier of Lieutenant-Colonel Ballard's by the grazing of a cannon shot, had a great part of his forehead carried off, and the skull fractured into many pieces, and some of it driven with the hairy scalp into the brain. The man fell down as dead, but after a while moved and an hour or two after, his fellow soldiers seeing him endeavour to rise, fetched me to him. I pulled out the pieces of bones and lacerated flesh from amongst the brain, in which they were entangled, and dressed him up with soft folded linen dipped in a Cephalick Balsam, and with emplaster and bandage, bound him up supposing I should never dress him any more. Yet he lived 17 days and the 15th day walked from that great corner fort over against Portland by the bridge which separates Weymouth from Melcomb-Regis only led by the hand of someone of his fellow soldiers. The second day after he fell into a spasmus, and died, howling like a dog as most of those do who have been so wounded. (This was presumably tetanus—HE).

At the siege of Taunton, one of Colonel John Arundell's men, in storming the works, was shot in the face by case-shot. He fell down, and in the retreat was carried off among the dead and laid into an empty house by the way until the next day; when in the morning early, the Colonel marching by that house heard a knocking within against the door. Some of the officers, desiring to know what it was, looked in, and saw this man standing by the door without eyes, face, nose or mouth. The Col. sent for me to dress the man. I went, but was somewhat troubled by where to begin . . . his face, with his eyes, nose, mouth and forepart of the jaw, with the chin, was shot away and the remaining parts of the them driven in. One part of the jaw hung down by his throat, and the other part passed into it. I saw the brain working out underneath the lacerated scalp on both sides between his ears and brows. I could not see any advantage he could have by my dressing . . . but I helped him to clear his throat, where was remaining the root of his tongue. I asked him if he would drink, making a sign by holding up a finger. He presently did the like, and immediately after held up both his hands, expressing his thirst. A soldier fetched some milk and brought in a little wooden dish to pour some of it down his throat . . . he held the root of his tongue down with the one hand, and with the other poured it down his throat (carrying his head backward), and so got down more than a quarter. After that I bound his wounds up. The dead were removed from vents to their graves, and fresh straw was fetched for him to lie upon, with an old blanket to cover him. It was in the summer. There we left that deplorable creature to lodge, and while we continued there, which was about 6 or 7 days, he was dressed by some of the surgeons with a fomentation made of vulnerary plants, with a little brandy wine in it, and with stupes of tow dipped in our common digestive. So we bound him up.'

References

Kirkup J. *On Wounds, of Gun Shot Wounds, of Fractures and Luxations by Richard Wiseman, Sergeant Surgeon to Charles II, a facsimile of Books V, VI and VII*. Bath, England: Kingsmead, 1977.
Longmore T. *Richard Wiseman—Surgeon and Sergeant—Surgeon to Charles II, A Biographical Study*. London: Longmans Green, 1891.

[15]

Thomas Eshelby

Above elbow amputation on
Admiral Nelson (1797)

To any Englishman with a sense of History, the most famous amputation was that performed on Horatio Nelson.

In April 1797, Admiral Nelson, then 38 years of age, planned to seize treasure ships in the harbour at Santa Cruz on Teneriffe, one of the Canary Islands. He set off in July with a fleet of four ships of the line, three frigates and a cutter, but unfavourable currents and severe storms deprived the landing of any hope of surprise. Not discouraged, Nelson himself lead an armada of rowing boats, which set out from their mother-ships on the night of July 24th. The plan was simple, it was to land on the harbour mole and rush the main square of the town. As the boats approached the mole at half past one in the morning, the waiting Spaniards opened a murderous fire of cannon and muskets and there were heavy losses. One of the first casualties was Nelson himself. As he scrambled out of his boat and reached with his right arm to draw his sword, a grape shot shattered his right humerus. 'I am shot through the arm, I am a dead man', he exclaimed.

Nelson's life was probably saved by his step-son Lieutenant Josiah Nisbet, who used his silk neckerchief to fashion a tourniquet around Nelson's arm, hoisted the wounded Admiral back onto the boat, seized one of the oars and helped row him back from the scene of carnage.

Nelson was rowed to his flagship, the 'Sea Horse', but refused to be carried on board. The reason for this extraordinary act was one of quite remarkable chivalry. Nelson knew that on the 'Sea Horse' was Betsy Fremantle, the pregnant wife of Nelson's captain. Nelson also knew that Fremantle was still somewhere on the beach and he refused to be seen by her in his wounded condition without being able to give her news of her husband (who was indeed wounded in the same action). Nelson insisted that he be rowed on to 'Theseus'. Here, he hoisted himself onto the deck and said 'Tell the surgeon to make haste and get his instruments. I know I must lose my right arm and the sooner it is off the better'.

The surgeon on 'Theseus' was Thomas Eshelby, then 28 years of age. His assistant was Louis Remonier, a 24 year old French Royalist refugee, who had trained at Toulon and was serving in the Royal Navy with the rank of surgeon's mate.

The amputation was carried out in the early hours of the morning of July 25th in the cold cockpit of 'Theseus'. The operation would have been performed by lamp light with the ship tossing on the waves and to the sounds of the groans of the other wounded.

Eshelby's log, from which this case report is copied, and which is still carefully preserved at the Public Records Office at Kew, records that Nelson was obviously the 'first on the operating list'. The other casualties dealt with that morning were:-

1. James Holden—Seaman—aged about 27; wounded breast, compound fracture of right arm close to the shoulder by a musket ball through the pectoral muscle and after through the arm dividing the humeral artery; immediate amputation.

2. John Wilson—Seaman—aged about 29, wound of breast and shoulder by musket ball passing through the breast and scapula; haemorrhage suppressed by compression.

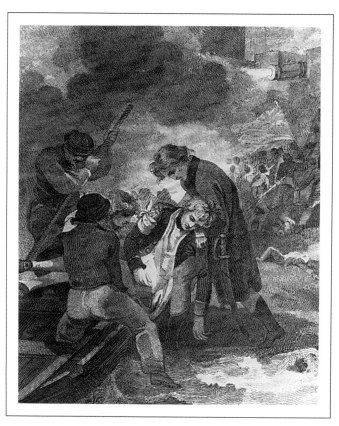

Nelson wounded at Teneriffe. Josiah Nisbet has used his own neckerchief as a tourniquet
(From *Orme's Graphic History of the Life, Exploits and Death of Horatio Nelson* London; Edward Orme 1806)

3. William Harrison—Seaman—aged about 30, compound fracture of left arm by a musket ball striking the radius, ball and several pieces of bone extracted.

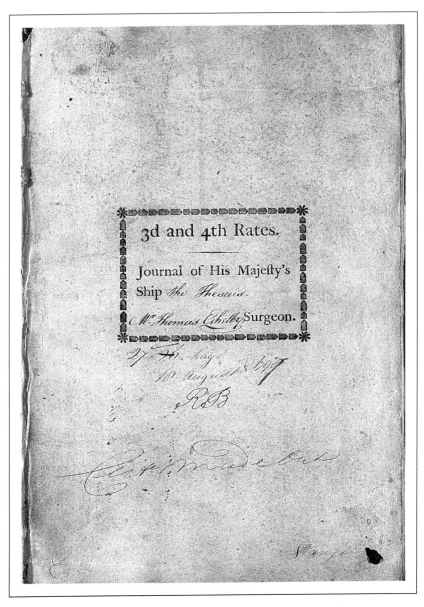

The front cover of Thomas Eshelby's log, HMS Theseus
(Reproduced with permission of the Public Record Office, Kew, Controller of Her Majesty's Stationery Office. Crown Copyright)

The entry in Eshelby's log for 25 July 1797. Nelson heads the list of casualties

(Reproduced with permission of the Public Record Office, Kew, Controller of Her Majesty's Stationery Office. Crown Copyright)

4. Lieutenant Weatherhead, aged about 22, wound of stomach by a ragged ball in great pain with violent vomiting of green and yellow fluids. (This unfortunate young man died five days later).

5. Thomas Kelly—marine—aged about 29, contusion of the side by a ball that fractured the ribs.

6. William Turner—wounded fingers.

Four further seamen were admitted with pain in the back, loins and limbs having been immersed for a long time in water when their cutter sank.

There was, of course, no anaesthesia. No doubt Nelson would have been given a tot of rum and a leather pad to bite upon but immediately post operatively he was given a stiff dose of opium. When asked if he wanted his limb embalmed, Nelson said 'throw it into the hammock with the brave fellow that was killed beside me'. (Dead sailors were sewn into their hammocks for burial at sea.)

Not a great deal is known about Thomas Eshelby, but there are some manuscript notes about him deposited in the library of the Royal College of Surgeons of England by Warren Dawson in 1933: Eshelby was born at Thirsk in Yorkshire on the 27th February 1769, he qualified at Surgeon's Hall in 1791 and was promoted to surgeon fourth rate in 1794. He joined 'Theseus' and opened his log on 27th May 1797 until he transferred to 'Sea Horse' on August 20th to accompany Nelson back to England.

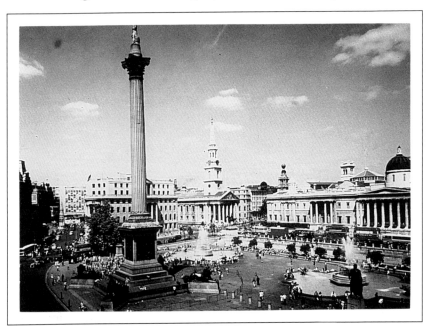

Nelson's column, Trafalgar Square, London

In 1801, Eshelby married Peggy Douglas, whose brother, Captain John Douglas R.N., curiously also had his arm amputated at Teneriffe. They had seven children, one of who became a naval surgeon and another a Lieutenant in the Royal Navy. Eshelby died at Plymouth on 19th February 1811, at the age of 41, being then surgeon on HMS Caton, and was buried at Stoke Damerel.

Nelson made a satisfactory recovery from his amputation. On the fifth post-operative day he required a dose of senna and Jalap and one wonders whether his constipation was due to his post-operative opium. However, there was a persistent sinus where the long silk ligature around the brachial artery emerged from the wound. In addition, the ligature almost certainly incorporated the median nerve, since Nelson experienced a great deal of pain in the stump. The ligature came away on the 3rd December, following which the sinus healed quickly and the pain was considerably relieved. On the 8th December, Nelson, who was then lodging in Bond Street, in London, sent a note to the vicar of St George's Hanover Square which stated 'An officer desires to return thanks to Almighty God for his perfect recovery from a severe wound, and also for many mercies bestowed upon him'.

When the bills came to be settled for the amputation, Thomas Eshelby received £36 and Louis Remonier 24 guineas for assistance at the operation and for sitting up a total of 14 nights with the patient.

Thomas Eshelby, Surgeon, "Journal of His Majesty's Ship The Theseus. 27 May–18 August 1797"

'Admiral Nelson, 25 July. Compound fracture of the right arm by a musket ball passing thro' a little above the elbow; an artery divided; the arm was immediately amputated and the following give him,
R. Opii gr. ij. f. Pil. statim s.
  Rep Pil Opii gr j
  Rep Pil Opii gr ij hora. s. s.

July 6. Rested pretty well and is quite easy.
Mist Salin oz ij ter in die
Repetr. Pil Opii hora.s.s.
Tea, Soup, Sago, Lemonade and Tamarind Drink.

July 27th. Had a middling night, no fever.
Rep. Pil Opii hora somni s.

July 28th. Dressed the stump, look'd well.
R Decoct Cinchona oz iss ter in die
Rep Pil Opii h.s.s.

July 29th. Pretty easy had no stool since the operation gave the following.
R Infus senae oz ij Pulv Jalap
Rep Pil Opii hora somni s.

July 30th. Cathartic operated well, pretty easy. Rep Pil h.s.s. Rep decoct Cinchona.

July 31st. One of the ligatures came away it looks well. Rep med ut heri.

August 1st. Continued getting well very fast, stump look'd well, no bad symptom whatever occurred, he continued the use of the Cortex and a gentle opening Draught occasionally.

Discharged on board the 'Sea Horse' 20th August. The sore reduced to the size of a shilling, in perfect good health one of the ligatures not come away.'

Glossary

Opii gr ij f. Pil. statim s. = Opium pill 2 grains; let it be taken at once.
Rep Pil Opii gr ij hora s.s. = Repeat opium pill 2 grains; let it be taken at the hour of sleep.
Mist Salin oz ij ter in die. = Saline mixture 2 fluid ounces three times a day. (Probably Bicarbonate of Potash.)
Decoct Cinchona oz iss. = Cinchona 1½ fluid ounces. (Quinine is derived from cinchona bark.)
Rep med ut heri = Repeat medicines as directed yesterday.
Bark = Cinchona bark (prescribed as a febrifuge).

Note
Professor John Trounce estimates that two grains of opium pill was probably equivalent to 6.5 mgm of morphia.

References

Dawson WE. *Thomas Eshelby (manuscript notes)*. Royal College of Surgeons of England library. Tracts B 1933 Volume 354.
Ellis H. *Famous Operations*. Media: Harwal, 1984.
Eshelby T. *Journal of His Majesty's Ship Theseus 27 May–18 August 1797*. Kew: Public Records Office.
Power D. Amputation: the operation on Nelson in 1797. *British Journal of Surgery*. 1932; **19**: 352–355.
Pugh PDG. *Nelson and His Surgeons*. Edinburgh: Livingstone, 1968.

[16]
Dominique Jean Larrey
Gunshot wounds of the bladder (1814)

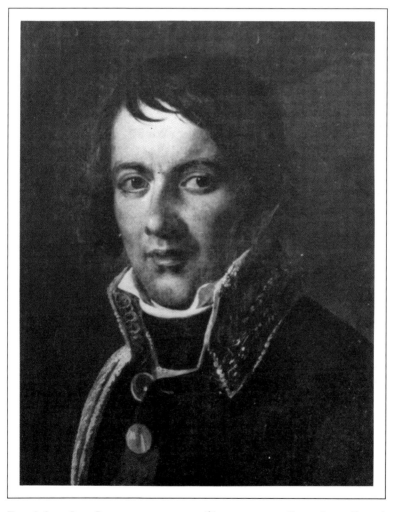

Dominique Jean Larrey as a young military surgeon. Portrait attributed
to Mme Benoit
(From J. Henry Dible *Napoleon's Surgeon*. London; Heinemann, 1970, with
permission of the publisher)

No one would argue that France has produced two of the world's greatest war surgeons—Ambroise Paré and Dominique Jean Larrey. We are fortunate that both of them have bequeathed to their surgical descendants extensive case reports which vividly portray their contributions to the surgery of the battle field.

Larrey was born in 1766 in a small village in the French Pyrenees. At the tender age of 13, he became apprenticed to his brother Alexis, a surgeon in Toulouse. On qualification, he joined the French navy in 1787 and served as ship's surgeon along the coasts of Newfoundland. He returned to France a few months before the Revolution of 1789.

In 1792, Larrey was posted to the Army of the Rhine and from then on was engaged in almost continuous active military duties until Waterloo in 1815, where he was seriously wounded; duties which took him all over Europe, Egypt, Syria and Russia in 25 campaigns and 60 battles. He was Chief Surgeon to the Imperial Guard, Surgeon in Chief to the Imperial Army and Professor of Surgery at the army medical school at Val-de-Grâce. He was created Baron by Napoleon after the Battle of Wagram in 1809.

After the Napoleonic wars, Larrey became Surgeon Inspector to the Army Health Council and Chief Surgeon at the Hôtel Des Invalides in Paris and thus continued to serve military medicine in his care of the army veterans until his retirement at the age of 72. He died in 1842, lies buried in Père Lachaise Cemetery and his statue by David is to be found in front of the military hospital at Val-de-Grâce.

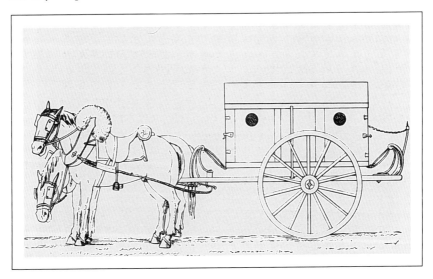

Larrey's 'Flying ambulance'.
(From J. Henry Dible *Napoleon's Surgeon*. London, Heinemann 1970, with permission of the publisher)

Larrey's contributions to military surgery were primarily his organizational skills in getting his surgical teams near the front line to ensure early surgery for the wounded and in stressing the rapid evacuation of wounded men by means of his specially designed light horse-drawn ambulances. His work was the foundation of the present day MASH concept.

The following case histories, from his account of the campaigns in Egypt and Syria, are typical of his vivid descriptive skills and wide experience of wartime trauma.

DJ Larrey "Memoirs of military surgery, and campaigns of the French armies"

First American edition, Baltimore: Joseph Cushing 1814, Volume 1, 321–4

'The case of Francis Chaumette, of the 22nd regiment of cavalry, who was wounded at the battle of Tabor, is the most remarkable. The ball passed through the hypogastrick region, across the pelvis, to that point of the left buttock, which is opposite the sciatick notch. The direction of the wound, and the escape of faecal matter and urine from both orifices, gave evidence that the bladder and rectum were injured. M. Milioz, who had the surgical direction of Kleber's division, carefully pursued the plan that had been adopted at Acre: the patient had fever when suppuration came on, and the pus was abundant, when the sloughs came away. A sound being introduced into the bladder, prevented the diffusion of urine, and facilitated the adhesion of the edges of the wounds of this viscus, which healed first. This man was perfectly well when he returned to Cairo.

I shall notice another case of Dacio, a corporal of the 9th demi-brigade, about 27 years of age, who was shot in the 11th assault on Acre. The ball went through the right buttock near the isciatick tuberosity, into the pelvis, and through the lower part of the bladder. The rectum was injured, and the ball came out in the perineum, where the operation of lithotomy is generally performed: it turned forward to the right, elevated a portion of the triceps femoris, and came out in the right groin near the crural arch, and on the inside of the crural vessels, which fortunately escaped unhurt.

The sudden discharge of urine through the inferior wounds, and the involuntary expulsion of faeces produced by the rupture of the sphincter ani, pointed out the injury of these organs. The patient suffered acute pain, and was uneasy, agitated, and in a state of insupportable tenesmus. The fever came on in the first twenty-four hours, and was very considerable until the eschars separated.

This man having been brought to my ambulance, I first attended to him, and continued to direct his treatment until he was cured. I first dilated the external wounds deeply, and the first day I passed an elastick sound into the bladder, to prevent the diffusion of urine I had a tent covered with cerate passed into the rectum; I prescribed clysters and a cooling regimen. At first he was very ill; when the sloughs came away on the ninth or tenth day, the symptoms abated: he passed but little urine through the wound, and seldom discharged faeces through it. The wound of the buttock healed first; then that of the groin: but that in the perineum did not heal until it had been under my direction six weeks, and entrusted to the particular care of my pupil, Mr Zink. He recovered entirely, and had neither incontinence of urine or faeces.

Desjardins, a fusilier of the 32nd demi brigade, was wounded in a sortie of the garrison of Acre, by a ball, which passed through the pelvis from the left sciatick notch, to the scrotum of the right side, where it lodged. The neck of the bladder was perforated at two opposite points, and the urine insinuated itself into the scrotum, which swelled prodigiously, and fell into gangrene. Mr Gallant, the surgeon, enlarged the wound by which the ball entered, and made an incision into the scrotum, where it had lodged. On the following day it was necessary to make deep scarifictions of these parts, to arrest the progress of the gangrene, and to assist nature in throwing off the slough; in the mean time he introduced a gum elastick sound into the bladder which prevented the subsequent diffusion of urine. After fifteen days of suffering, he began to improve; the eschars separated, the posterior wound soon closed, but that of the scrotum continued a long time open. When we returned to Egypt, a urinary fistula still remained, but healed soon after this period.

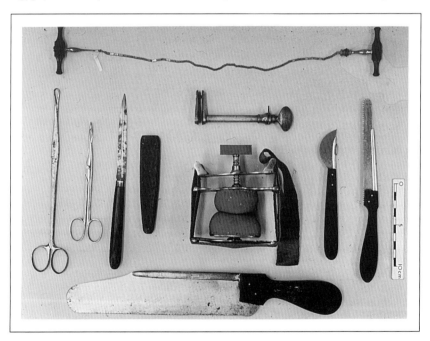

A selection of surgical instruments used by Baron Larrey.
(Wellcome Institute Library, reproduced with permission of the Wellcome Institute, London)

Many other similar cases occurred in the different engagements which we have since had, and all the wounded recovered by the same treatment. General Bon alone died of a wound of this kind, because he would not permit the wounds to be dilated, nor a sound to be introduced into the bladder. The diffusion of urine soon produced a gangrene, which was promoted by the corpulency of the general.'

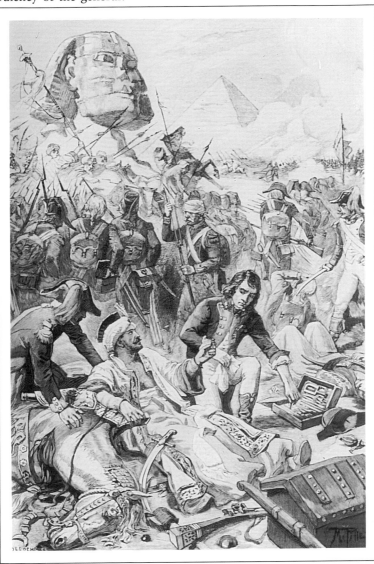

Larrey on the Battlefield, Battle of the Pyramids, 1798.
(From P. Triaire *Napoléon et Larrey* Tours: A. Mame 1902, Wellcome Institute Library, reproduced with permission of the Wellcome Institute, London)

References

Dible JH. *Napoleon's Surgeon* London: Heinemann, 1970

Larrey DJ. *Memoirs of Military Surgery and Campaigns of the French Armies.* 1st American edition, Baltimore; Joseph Cushing, 1814; Volume I: 321–3.

[17]

George Grey Turner

A bullet in the heart (1917)

The heart was long regarded as a surgical 'no go' area. Wounds of the heart were thought to be fatal and certainly beyond the help of the surgeon. Indeed, it was not until 1897 that Ludwig Rehn of Frankfurt am Main performed the first successful repair of a cardiac injury and even in the First World War such operations were rarities. George Grey Turner was a pioneer in many fields of surgical endeavour and it comes as no surprise that he performed one of the early operations (albeit unsuccessful), for a cardiac foreign body.

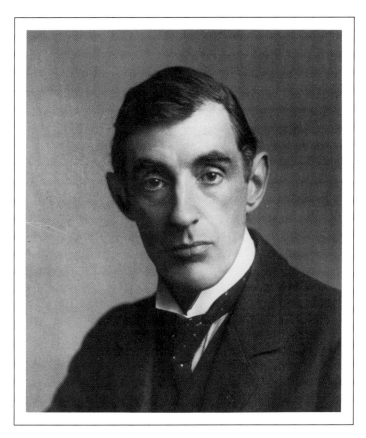

George Grey Turner
(Reproduced by permission of the President and Council of the Royal College of Surgeons of England)

Grey Turner was the son of a Newcastle banker. He attended the Medical School of the University of Durham and qualified with First Class Honours in 1898, proceeding to his FRCS in 1903. After working at King's College Hospital and Vienna, he returned to Newcastle, to his revered chief, Rutherford Morison. Soon promoted to the staff of the Royal Victoria Infirmary, he built up an immense surgical practice throughout Northumberland.

In 1914, he was called up as a Territorial and sent as a Colonel to the Middle East, before being made Consultant Surgeon to the Northern Command in England. It was in this capacity that he performed the cardiac operation reported below.

In 1927, Grey Turner was appointed Professor of Surgery in Newcastle, leaving there to be the first Director of Surgery at the newly opened Post-graduate Medical School in Hammersmith, where he served from 1934 to 1945. His interests ranged over the whole field of general surgery, but he was particularly well known for his radical operations for advanced abdominal cancer, for the surgery of the oesophagus, (he was one of the first to perform a successful oesophagectomy for cancer), and for the surgery of congenital defects of the bladder.

As a medical student in Oxford in 1945, the author was privileged to attend several of Grey Turner's clinical demonstrations. He was a small man with a large head (on the back of which he would usually perch a bowler hat). He paid little attention to his appearance, wore shabby clothes and old boots, which he repaired himself. He spoke with a Northumberland accent, but he mesmerized we young students by his enthusiasm and pithy aphorisms. He told us 'you are not a surgeon until you have operated upon a strangulated hernia on a kitchen table by candlelight'. Actually, I have personally never done this, although I have performed a Ramstedt operation in a bathroom by an Anglepoise lamp!

George Grey Turner died suddenly in 1951 at the age of 73.

G Grey Turner "A bullet in the heart for twenty-three years"

Lancet 1940; ii: 487–489

'A general interest in the fate of foreign bodies encourages me to report the case of a man who is alive and well and has gone about his daily work for the last 23 years with a bullet lodged in the wall of the left ventricle.

The patient, aged 32, was admitted to a base hospital under my care in April 1917. 18 days before admission he was struck on the front of the left side of the chest by a bullet from a machine gun at an estimated range of 500 yards. There was also a through-and-through wound of the left arm just above the elbow; this may have been inflicted by the same bullet which penetrated the chest. In its course the missile traversed a service waterproof, the left breast pocket of his tunic with its contents and his shirt.

When I first saw the patient, his only complaint was of some slight soreness about the wound on the chest. He was a well-developed man with rather a big chest and looked fit and well. There was a small wound of entrance ¼in. below and ¼in. external to the left nipple, but there was no wound of exit. There were the scars of the through-and-through wound 2 in. above the left elbow, but this had apparently done no damage, and no disability ever arose from it. The situation of the wound on the chest wall at once

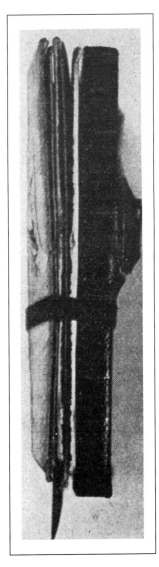

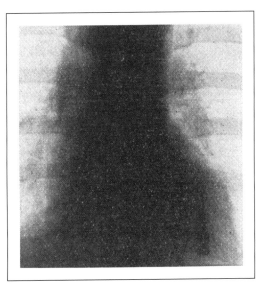

Radiogram showing bullet in left ventricle
twenty years after the casualty
(Reproduced by permission of the *Lancet*)

(left) Notebook and letters traversed by bullet
before entering the heart
(Reproduced by permission of the *Lancet*)

suggested the possibility of some cardiac injury, but there were no characteristic signs. The pulse was regular and its average rate 64 and the temperature was normal. There was no dyspnoea.

Radiography showed that a service bullet, with its base anchored probably near the tip of the left ventricle, was pulsing with the heart beat, while its point was whirled about in the blood vortex in the heart cavity. An electrocardiogram was submitted to the late Sir James Mackenzie, who reported:-

> The electrocardiogram shows nothing peculiar, excepting in the second lead where the wave T is inverted. This inversion of T was assumed at one time to be of serious significance, but I have watched cases who show it for a great many years and this view has turned out to be unjustified.

The patient was apparently quite well and was finding enforced rest irksome. On May 12 he was allowed to get up and to walk about the ward and up and down stairs.

Operation

It seemed that the patient ran a great risk with a foreign body in so precarious a position, and I feared that at some time it would become dislodged and cause fatal embolism, or that blood would clot about it and produce a thrombus which might also cause embolism. Consequently, I decided to remove the bullet.

The operation was performed on May 20, thirty-nine days after the receipt of the wound. The anaesthetic used was A.C.E. followed by open ether. The approach was made by the left parasternal route, and the general technique was as described by Theodore Kocher, in the third English edition of his textbook of operative surgery.

The skin incisions were along the line of the left sixth costal cartilage and vertically over the sternum to the level of the second. As a first step the 6th costal cartilage was excised and the pericardium easily exposed by dividing the attachment of the triangularis sterni muscle along the seventh costal cartilage and the sternum and pushing it outwards and upwards. Immediately air began to be sucked into the cellular tissue around the pericardium to such an extent that this area rapidly became emphysematous. It closely simulated air in the pleura and was rather an anxiety throughout the operation, though it was controlled to some extent by covering up the exposed part with large wet gauze swabs. The fifth and fourth costal cartilages were next cleared, the pleura being separated from their deep surfaces and gently pushed outwards by the finger before they were divided.

The flap of chest wall was then bent outwards; but, since this did not give enough working space, the third cartilage also was cut through and displaced. The pericardium, which was not distended, was readily opened by an oblique incision about 2 inches long made in the direction of the sixth cartilage. A little bloodstained fluid escaped, but there were no clots and no adhesions. When the heart was first exposed, it beat in a tremulous fashion, but soon quietened down, and throughout the subsequent manipulation its movements were steady.

The spot where the bullet had entered, about the middle of the outer border of the left ventricle slightly towards its posterior aspect, was marked by a depression surrounded by a roughened whitish area on the visceral pericardium. . . . The left auricle was then explored by external palpation, but nothing abnormal was detected.

It was still felt that the bullet might be lodged about the suspected area near the base of the ventricle. To steady the heart for final exploration a stitch of fine catgut was passed into the wall of the ventricle just by the side of the entrance scar. To gain a little more working space the sternal stumps of the divided costal cartilages were removed. Gentle traction on the stitch steadied this portion of the heart wall without in the least affecting its general action. Further punctures were made with the needle, but no bullet was found.

Since I was reluctant to give up the attempt, I exposed the posterior surface of the heart high up behind the ventricle by rotating the heart and then taking it into my hand for thorough palpation. By this method something hard and elongated could be felt in the centre of the heart, presumably near the base of the inter-ventricular septum. But this examination gave us a fright, because the heart stopped beating as soon as mild pressure was applied to the base.

Consequently the heart was replaced in its normal position and the pericardium was sutured, a small drainage-tube being left in the lowest part of the sac and another laid along the outside near the suture line. The flap of chest was replaced and held in position with catgut sutures between the periosteum of the sternum and the perichondral structures. The skin was sutured with interrupted silkworm without tension, the drains being brought through the centre of the lower oblique incision.

The operation took an hour and three-quarters, the greater part of that time being spent in efforts to locate the bullet. The patient stood the ordeal well and immediate recovery was satisfactory. The only troublesome symptom was persistent vomiting without nausea, and this was really distressing. For days the patient could keep nothing down, but in spite of this he seemed well and was quiet and undisturbed. In the course of a week the condition gradually subsided, having been entirely uninfluenced by treatment. The patient was well enough to be out of bed in three weeks. Five weeks, the wound was firmly consolidated and the chest expanding well. Radiography a month after the operation showed the bullet in precisely the same position as before and moving with the heart beat, but the whirling movement has ceased.

Subsequent history

The patient left hospital nine weeks after the operation and thereafter steadily improved. In November he reported himself as very well, and next year he was transferred to the records office of his regiment. After taking his discharge early in 1922 he had a long rest after which he was able to do all ordinary things in moderation, including a mild game of golf. Ten years after the operation he married. At times he was perhaps rather apprehensive and a little too careful. In consequence, he put on weight unduly and suffered from indigestion.

In June 1937, i.e., just over twenty years after the wound, he came to see me. He was very well and had no cardiac disability. His employment was indoors, but he lived in the country and usually drove his car to his office seven miles from home. . . . He had given up golf a few years ago because he thought it would perhaps be wiser not to exert himself unduly. Five years ago his appendix was removed under local anaesthesia. Recovery was uneventful and he was back at the office in five weeks.

Dr Duncan White radiographed him and reported 'a bullet is embedded in the wall of the left ventricular septum. Its movement is synchronous with

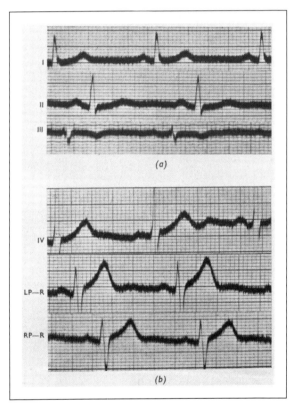

(a)

(b)

Electrocardiograms taken twenty years after bullet
entered heart: (a) limb leads (b) chest leads
(Reproduced by permission of the *Lancet*)

the cardiac contractions. There is slight enlargement and rounding of the left ventricle, with very slight unfolding of the aorta'. . . .

In April 1940, the patient reported that he was quite well, though he confessed to being a little tired, 'a result of the present war, not the last one!'. When fatigued he suffers from what he describes as indigestion, but this passes off after a week or ten days' rest.

Conclusion

The management of cases of foreign body in the heart which are not immediately fatal must be settled on general surgical principles. Nature should be assisted to exhibit her powers as a healer, and the patient with cardiac disability after gunshot wound should have many months of rest. If, in spite of a fair chance, the disability persists or develops after a period and interferes with usefulness, the aid of surgery may properly be invoked; but the difficulties may be very great, and even during operation a wise restraint may save a disaster. As the late Mr Frank Jeans of Liverpool was fond of saying 'A living problem is better than a dead certainty'.

References

Grey Turner G. A bullet in the heart for twenty three years. *Lancet* 1940; **2**: 487–9.
Wakeley C. (Editor) *Great teachers of Surgery of the Past*. A collection of articles which have appeared in the *British Journal of Surgery* over the period January 1964 to January 1968. Bristol: Wright, 1969; 135–140.

[18]

Harvey Cushing

Gunshot wounds of the head (1917)

Harvey Cushing (1869–1939) founded a school of neurosurgery, first at the
Johns Hopkins Hospital, Baltimore, and then at the Brigham Hospital,
Boston, whose disciples are now found throughout the world. His contributions
to the elective surgery of the brain are well known. His clinical contributions
included the description of Cushing's syndrome, his monograph on pituitary
tumours, his meticulous documentation of more than 2000 verified cerebral
tumours, and his introduction of the diathermy and haemostatic clips, which
greatly reduced the blood loss during cerebral operations.

He trained many of the men who themselves became pioneers in this
demanding field, including Walter Dandy, Gilbert Horrax, Ernest Sachs and
an Australian, Hugh Cairns, who subsequently became my Professor of

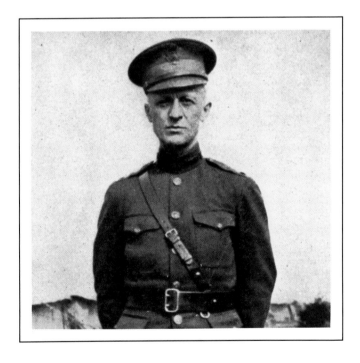

Harvey Cushing
(From H. Cushing, *From a Surgeon's Journal* London, Constable
1936, reproduced with permission of the publisher)

Surgery in Oxford. The author can therefore claim, with the greatest diffidence, to be a third generation Cushing man!

Less well recognized, perhaps, is Cushing's important work on the management of penetrating injuries of the skull and brain. This includes his rotation flap for closure of scalp defects, the use of the sucker to debride cerebral wounds and the electromagnet to remove metallic foreign bodies from the brain.

Most of his experience in war wounds of the head came from his periods of intensive military service in World War I. In the Spring of 1915, he served with a Harvard unit at Neuilly, where he dealt with French casualties. On his return to USA, he realized that American intervention in the war was inevitable and set about the organization of a Base Hospital in Boston. He was sent to France again in May 1917, attached to the British Expeditionary Force, and, in June 1918, he became Senior Consultant in Neurosurgery to the American Expeditionary Force. He dealt with the casualties from the three major engagements which involved American troops—Château-Thierry, St Mihiel and the Argonne.

Throughout this period of military service, Cushing kept a meticulous, almost daily diary, much of it written on the back of used temperature charts, X-ray reports and other scraps of paper. Often these were written late at night or while being driven in an ambulance. His diary eventually filled nine bound volumes in his own library.

The Cushing family, on the paternal side, originated from Gravesend, England. Matthew Cushing, a deacon, emigrated to Boston in 1638. Harvey was preceded by three generations of doctors, his father practised in Cleveland, Ohio in Obstetrics. Harvey's mother came of pioneer mid-western stock.

Cushing was educated at Yale and at Harvard Medical School, Boston. While still a medical student, Cushing gave his first indication of his genius for clinical innovation. It was the practice in those days for clinical students to be responsible for the administration of anaesthesia. Together with his class-mate, Amory Codman, Cushing devised the first anaesthetic chart in 1894. Several years later, he incorporated blood pressure measurements on his chart during all major operations.

Cushing qualified in 1895 and was appointed to the House Staff at the Massachusetts General Hospital, Boston. Here he and Codman again collaborated, this time on the clinical use of X-rays, whose discovery had only been made by Röntgen in the December of the previous year.

In the Autumn of 1896, at the age of 27, Cushing became Assistant Resident to William Stewart Halsted at the Johns Hopkins Hospital in Baltimore. After a period of study in Europe, Cushing was drawn more and more into the field of neurosurgery, with particular emphasis on cranial tumours and on diseases of the pituitary body. However, it was not until 1932 that he described the basophil tumour of the pituitary associated with the syndrome that now carries his name.

In 1910, at the age of 41, Cushing accepted the Chair of Surgery at Harvard Medical School and at the end of 1912, moved to Boston into the newly built Peter Bent Brigham Hospital.

After his army service, alluded to above, his services with the British Army having been recognized by the award of a Companion of the Bath, Cushing returned to his extensive clinical practice in Boston. As well as this, in 1920, shortly after the death of his old friend Sir William Osler, Cushing was approached by Lady Osler to write his biography. This was published in two volumes and 1413 pages in 1925. Amazingly, although an intimate friend of Osler for some 20 years, Cushing himself never mentions his own name throughout the biography, even to the extent of not stating that he had attended Osler's son, Revere, when he was fatally wounded in France in 1917. For this magnificent work, Cushing was awarded the Pullitzer Prize for 1926.

In 1931, Cushing operated upon his 2000th verified brain tumour and retired the following year. Cushing died in October 1939, at the age of 70, of a myocardial infarction.

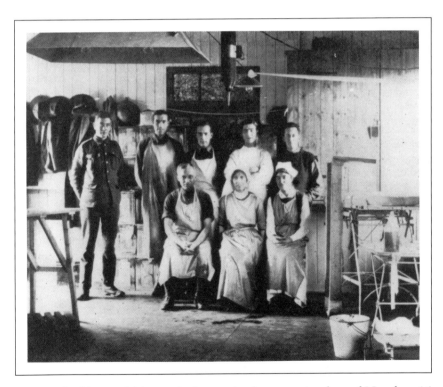

Harvey Cushing and his surgical team in the operating hut of Number 46 Casualty Clearing Station. Cushing is seated on the left of the two nurses. (From H. Cushing, *From a Surgeon's Journal* London, Constable 1936, reproduced with permission of the publisher)

In 1936, Cushing edited his war diaries into a single volume, now long out of print. Today, his case reports read with great poignancy and illustrate, perhaps as well as any written account by any other surgical author, the horrors and futility of war.

Harvey Cushing "From a surgeon's journal 1915–1918"

London: Constable, 1936

'Wednesday, August 15 (1917)

We nearly 'busted' on six cases in the twenty four hours since yesterday's note. We began at 8 pm on 'L/Cpl Wiseman 392332; 1/9 Londons SW Frac Skull', which interpreted means that a lance corporal of the 9th Londons had a shell wound. It went through his helmet in the parietal region, with indriven fragments to the ventricle. These cases take a long time if done carefully enough to forestall infection, and it was eleven o'clock before we got to 'Sgt Chave, C. 25912, MGC 167-SW head and back-penet' according to his field ambulance card. This sergeant of the Machine Gunners had almost the whole of his right frontal lobe blown out, with a lodged piece of shell almost an inch square, and extensive radiating fractures, which mean taking off most of his frontal bone, including the frontal sinuses—an enormous operation done under local anaesthesia. We crawled home for some eggs in the mess and to bed at 2.30 am—six hours for these two cases.

Thursday, August 16

This morning a man named Ward, rifleman of the 10th Brigade, was ticketed for us in the Resuscitation Ward—hard to tell whether he or we were more unfit for operation. We began at 9 am—an hour earlier than we had ever succeeded in starting before, for there is always trouble in getting boiling water, owing to the scarcity of Primus stoves, so-called. A penetrating wound of occiput, with complete blindness, and lodgement of the missile in the right frontal lobe. Also with novocaine, lasting another three hours, with extraction of fragments driven into the ventricle. Saunders, with a mid-vertex wound, rigid extremities, unconscious, and two foreign bodies with many fragments of deeply embedded bone showing in the X-rays. This carried Morton and me up to 2.30—too late for lunch. I got what might be called a high tea, and Horrax, who had been recording cases and doing dressings, took Morton's place and we did two more penetrating cases and then our more serious dressings, and managed to get to the mess for dinner nearly on time.

They shove the more serious cases on to us, which is what we want, but I'm beginning to be a little doubtful about eight a day if they are all of this magnitude.

This has been an ordinary slack time with a 'take' of only 200 cases in rotation with our neighbours Nos 64 and 12. The rush has not yet come—another postponement: perhaps due to the heavy rains today.

Friday, August 17

We beat our record today with eight cases—all serious ones. A prompt start at 9 am with two cases always in waiting—notes made, X-rays taken, and heads shaved. It's amusing to think that at home I used to regard a single major cranial operation a day's work. These eight averaged two hours apiece—one or two very interesting ones. One in particular—a sergeant, unconscious, with a small wound of entrance in the vertex and a foreign body just beside the sella turcica. We have learned a new way of doing these things—viz., to encircle the penetrating wound in the skull with Montenovesi forceps, and to take the fractured area with the depressed bone fragments out in one piece—then to catheterize the tract and to wash it out with a Carrel syringe through the tube. In doing so the suction of the bulb is enough occasionally to bring out a small bone fragment clinging to the eye of the catheter. Indeed, one can usually detect fragments by the feel of the catheter, they are often driven in two or three inches.

In this particular man, however, after the tract was washed clear of blood and disorganized brain, the nail was inserted its full six inches and I tried twice unsuccessfully to draw out the fragment with the magnet. On the third attempt I found to my disgust that the current was switched off. There was nothing to do but make the best of it, and a small stomach tube was procured, cut off, boiled, inserted in the six inch tract, suction put on, and a deformed shrapnel ball (not the expected piece of steel shell) was removed on the first trial—of course a non-magnetizable object.

Tonight while operating on a Boche prisoner with a 'GSW head' about 11 pm—our seventh case—some Fritz planes came over on a bombing raid, as they do almost every night nowadays—nowanights (which is it?). Of course, all our lights were switched off, and we had to finish with candles. If we didn't do a very good job, it was Fritz's fault, not entirely ours.

The Boche prisoner, I may add, was a big fellow with a square head, badly punctured though it was. The case in waiting was a little eighteen year old Tommy from East London—scared, peaked, underfed, underdeveloped. He had been in training six months and was in the trenches for the first time during the present show—just ten minutes when he was hit.

Sunday, August 19

Morning

My prize patient, Baker, with the shrapnel ball removed from near his sella, after doing well for three days suddenly shot up a temperature to 104 last night about midnight. I took him to the operating theatre, reopened the perfectly healed external wounds, and found to my dismay a massive gas infection of the brain. I bribed two orderlies to stay up with him in the operating room, where he could have constant thorough irrigation over the brain and through the track of the missile. No light except candles was permitted last night. We fortunately are not taking in, and I was dressing him this morning, for he still lives, when someone leaning out of the window cried out 'There's a falling plane!'. Nose down, spinning, wings laid back, like a dead bird. He fell just beyond No. 64 and the familiar, irresistible impulse made everyone run toward the spot, I too as soon as I could leave. I got across the track, past the post-mortem tent, as far as the rapidly growing cemetery on the other side of No 64. Here were about a hundred grinning Chinese coolies, in their blue tunics, though some were stripped to the waist, digging two fresh ditches, about six by twenty feet. The Far East digging in the upstart West with its boasted civilization! This held me up, and I refrained from crossing the road to see the mangled machine and the dead thing under it.

Afternoon

Welpley has had the grass cut on the tennis court and the lines freshly marked out. He has arranged too, for a tournament, mixed doubles. We are to have tea served there. I am contributing a box of Page and Shaw's chocolates from the usual source of home comforts and delicacies.

Night, 11 pm

A baby crying in the operating theatre with a badly wounded arm; its mother on the next table with several small wounds and badly shocked. An unusual sight for a CCS. There had been the usual raid, one comes every evening. It's about our turn, and not a light is permitted. Rumour has it that these are reprisals, that one of our big naval guns fired into Roulers and hit a German hospital. Consequently, Rémy has had it, also Brandhoek, and yesterday Dosinghem, where there were many casualties, I believe, one of Brewer's American nurses was slightly wounded and some MO's also.

At ten or thereabouts, he came, a clear, cloudless, dark night with no moon, just right for him. We could get some idea of where he was by the focusing of the searchlights and where the Archies were bursting as they tried to pick him up. Twenty or more shafts, and in addition the two huge beams, from naval searchlights in Dunkerque, it is said, which simply poured shafts of light down in this direction. Once we saw him picked up with all the shafts for miles around focusing on him, but he dodged away. This was to the east of us, then Archies to the south in three places, so that possibly there was more than one raider, then after a time to the north, Bandagehem way, apparently, where he dropped eight bombs. The big French searchlights got at him and one heard machine gun fire, perhaps from Fritz himself. Finally, we could hear his engine as he passed over us, then two more explosions, and the searchlights began to blink off. He'd gone.

Then the baby and its mother, a *poilu*, and an excited Belgian, in the reception hut. Weird sight it was, candlelight, bearers and MO's in their tin hats, a wounded woman and her baby, the fruit of the raid.

Monday, August 20: midnight

A busy day. Six only, but one of them required three major operations, two cranial penetrations, one in the temporal, another in the vertex, and a bad shoulder wound as well. So this should count for eight. It was not our rotation, but Miller thought I had better take him on. All three were done under local anaesthesia, and during their course I learned from the man, whose name is Atkins, that he is a collier at home, a stretcher-bearer here. He had gone out to get a wounded man they had seen lying out for six days in a bad spot. No one else would go and finally volunteered, though the man didn't belong to his Division. That's all he remembers, though he was quite conscious tonight and can talk, for it's his right brain that's damaged. Hero? Not at all. It was only in the day's work, and probably no one will ever know or care. A simple coal miner.'

References

Cushing H. *From a Surgeon's Journal, 1915–1918*. London: Constable, 1936.
Fulton JF. *Harvey Cushing. A Biography*. Oxford: Blackwell, 1946.
Ellis H. Harvey Cushing. *Journal of Medical Biography* 1994; **2**: 71–77.

[19]

Gordon Gordon-Taylor

Gun shot wounds of the abdomen in war (1918)

Conservative treatment of gun shot wounds of the abdomen dominated the teachings of military surgeons in the American Civil War, the Franco-Prussian War of 1870–1871 and the Boer War of 1899–1902. This conservative approach was adopted at the beginning of World War I, but the mortality was frightful and amounted to about 80% at base hospitals. Many more victims, of course, died in the dressing stations along the lines of evacuation. Impressed by these awful results, a group of young British surgeons, operating at Casualty Clearing Stations close behind the front line, were able to show that early intervention gave the patients with gun shot wounds of the belly their only reasonable chance of survival. The first notable success was that of Owen Richards, a Professor of Surgery who had been made a temporary Captain in the British Expeditionary Force. Early in 1915 he performed two successful resections for gun shot wounds of the small intestine, one of 2½ and the second of 4½ feet of bowel. It was soon evident that early surgery was more or less the only hope for such cases. Even then, of course, in the

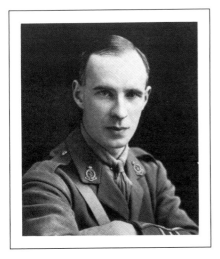 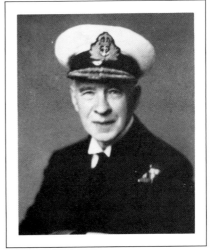

Gordon Gordon-Taylor, a Major in the RAMC in 1914   Gordon Gordon-Taylor, a Surgeon Rear-Admiral in 1940

(Reproduced with permission of the Director of Administrative Services, University College, London)

absence of antibiotics, effective fluid replacement and paucity of blood transfusions, the mortality remained high.

One of those young British surgeons was Major Gordon Gordon-Taylor. He was born in London in 1878, but on his father's death, the family moved to Aberdeen. At the age of 20 he took his degree in classics at Aberdeen University, and maintained his interest in the ancient languages all his life—his lectures often being studded with classical quotations, especially from his beloved Horace. He trained at the Middlesex Hospital, obtained a 1st class BSc in Anatomy, (another of his life-long loves), and, at the age of 29, was appointed to the staff of the Middlesex as Assistant Surgeon.

On the outbreak of war, Gordon-Taylor joined the Royal Army Medical Corps and his speed and skill, particularly in the surgery of abdominal and even thoraco-abdominal gun shot wounds became a legend. He served mainly in France, with No 5 CCS (Casualty Clearing Station) and dealt with the wounded of the Somme and Passchendale. He ended the war as Consultant Surgeon to the Fourth Army and was appointed an Officer of the British Empire in 1919.

After the war, Gordon-Taylor returned to the Middlesex and became an exponent of major surgery, particularly for cancer and for gastric haemorrhage. He performed no less than 100 hind quarter amputations.

At the outbreak of World War II, at the age of 61, Gordon-Taylor was dismayed to be turned down by the Army. However, he joined the Naval Medical Service as a Lieutenant and was immediately promoted Rear-Admiral. His experience and advice were invaluable, particularly in the management of air-raid casualties. He was knighted for his services in 1946.

Gordon-Taylor continued to lecture, teach and write until his death in 1960 as a result of being knocked down by a car as he walked away from a cricket match at Lord's. He was 82 years of age.

The following extract, from a little book he published at the outbreak of the Second World War, is characacteristic of Gordon Gordon-Taylor's dramatic style.

Gordon Gordon-Taylor "The abdominal injuries of warfare"

Bristol: Wright, 1939

'**Penetrating wound of the abdomen; hernia of the small bowel; wound of the bladder; fracture of rib, anterior portion of iliac crest, and pubic bone; double resection of the bowel; recovery.**

Private T was admitted into a casualty clearing station on September 18th 1918, with a severe wound of the abdomen. He came to operation eight and a half hours after being hit, and was found to have a hernia of shattered, strangled small intestine through a wound in the right hypochondrium; about 18 inches of bowel was thus prolapsed. The missile had then passed down between the internal oblique and transversalis muscles of the abdominal wall on the right side, and had struck against and shattered the anterior part of the crest of the ilium. Thence its course was deflected again into the peritoneal cavity, and it had become impacted in the posterior surface of the right pubic bone, transfixing the bladder and impaling a coil of ileum against that bone. With such force had the projectile been driven into the os pubis, that a considerable pull was required to dislodge it. The patient, when placed on the operating table, had a surprisingly good pulse of 96; but immediately the wound of entry was enlarged and the constriction of the neck of the prolapsed bowel thereby released, the pulse-rate rose to 130. The wound was filthy, and parietes and bowel alike were covered with grease and dirt. Four feet of badly damaged and perforated jejunum were resected, and other coils of jejunum and upper ileum were assiduously cleansed of grease and clothing. The coil of lower ileum impaled against the pubic bone was gangrenous and stinking, and a second resection of 2½ ft was performed. The posterior wall of the bladder was sutured and a glove drain was passed down into the cave of Retzius towards the wound on the anterior vesical surface. Very wide excision of the damaged abdominal muscles was performed, after the peritoneum had been closed; a defect in the latter was filled in by a graft of fascia obtained from the anterior layer of the sheath of the rectus. The anterior end of the crest of the ilium was widely exsected, the wound was packed with gauze soaked in flavine, and frequent instillations with flavine through Carrel's tubes were enjoined. A transfusion of 900 cc of blood was given and the patient was treated by the usual resuscitatory measures. The gauze and Carrel's tubes were removed on the fifth day and the skin was resutured. The patient was evacuated to the Base on the fourteenth day, and subsequently to England, February 7th 1919. Nearly 21 years later he is in good health.

Penetrating wound of the abdomen, severe wound of caecum and ascending colon; excision of caecum, ascending colon, and hepatic flexure; end-to-side union of ileum and transverse colon; suture of jejunum.

Private JK of the 1st Buffs, was admitted on November 20th 1917, into a Casualty Clearing Station with two penetrating wounds of the abdomen. Two

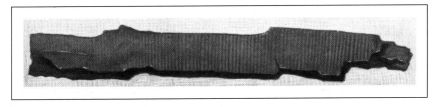

Private T. Fragment of high explosive, weighing 3 oz., which produced injuries to the abdominal wall and viscera, necessitating a double resection of bowel (× 4/5)

(From G. Gordon-Taylor *The Abdominal Injuries of Warfare* Bristol, Wright 1939)

fragments of shell had entered the abdominal cavity through the right flank, and the caecum and ascending colon were both badly damaged and perforated, the latter being almost completely divided. There were four wounds of the jejunum, which were sutured. Operation was performed about ten hours after the man was hit, and at the time he was in poor condition. The wounds in the flank were widely excised and subsequently vigorously treated with antiseptics; the terminal part of the ileum the caecum, ascending colon and hepatic flexure were excised and an end-to-side junction performed between the ileum and transverse colon. The patient made a good recovery, and was evacuated to England.

Penetrating wound of abdomen; resection of jejunum; end-to-end union; resection of distal part of transverse colon, splenic flexure, and descending colon; end-to-end union; caecostomy.

Lance-Corporal W of the MGC was admitted into a casualty clearing station in the early hours of a February morning 1918, with a penetrating wound of the abdomen produced by a shell fragment. The piece of shell entered the left flank, completely dividing his descending colon and shattering its adjacent edges. The upper jejunum was the site of several large perforations, and its mesentery was perforated and bleeding; 3 ft of jejunum was resected and an end-to-end junction performed. The missile had made a large rent on the posterior aspect of his transverse colon, and passing forwards and to the right half just penetrated the anterior surface of this portion of the bowel. It was deemed safer to excise the damaged portion of the transverse colon, splenic flexure, descending and iliac colon, and an end-to-end junction was performed between the proximal portion of the transverse colon and the sigmoid. The wound of entry was excised widely and 'Carrelled'; a temporary caecostomy was then performed. Apart from passive collapse of the lower lobe of his left lung and some trouble with the laparotomy wound, the patient made a good recovery, and was evacuated to the base a month later and subsequently to England.

Penetrating wound of abdomen; resection of small bowel and of sigmoid.

Private GW was admitted into a casualty clearing station in the early hours of a January morning 1918, with a penetrating wound of the abdomen, due to a fragment of shell. After the patient had been warmed and resuscitated for a couple of hours, the abdomen was opened, and nine or ten perforations of the jejunum were sutured, and in addition 18 in of small intestine lower down was resected. Four wounds of the sigmoid were found, two of which were on the mesenteric border; as the bowel was in a state of infarction, the damaged portion was resected and an end-to-end junction made. The foreign body was removed from the musculature of the left flank, and the damaged tissues widely excised; a temporary caecostomy was performed. The patient's recovery was uneventful; the caecostomy closed after ten days, by which time the rectum was acting satisfactorily, and he was evacuated to the base in three weeks, and subsequently to England.'

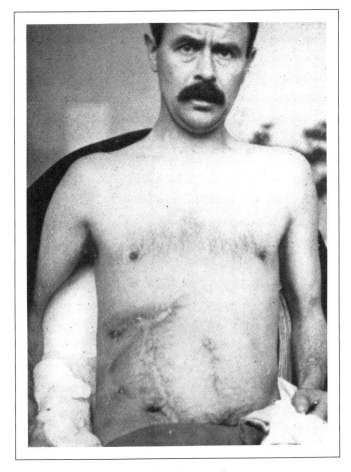

Private T, 20 years later
(From G. Gordon-Taylor *The Abdominal Injuries of Warfare*
Bristol, Wright 1939)

Notes on abbreviations

1st Buffs—the first battalion of a famous English infantry regiment.
MGC—Machine Gun Corps.

References

Gordon-Taylor G. *The Abdominal Injuries of Warfare*. Bristol: John Wright and Sons, 1939.
Hobsley M. Sir Gordon Gordon-Taylor: a biography and an appreciation. *Journal of Medical Biography* 1993; **1**: 83–9.

[20]

Anonymous

Civilian injuries from bombing (1941, 1942)

Although bombings of civilian targets were common enough in the Spanish Civil War and during the Italian invasion of Ethiopia, it was the Second World War that saw the horrors of aerial warfare spread across much of the civilized world. The names of London, Coventry, Merseyside, Rotterdam, Warsaw, Leningrad and Dresden are among the many cities that come to mind at once to anyone who lived through those dark and dangerous days.

The doctors who had to deal with civilian bomb casualties in the United Kingdom had none of the glamour of military uniforms and service ranks enjoyed by the young and fit members of the profession. They included general practitioners over military age, surgeons called out of retirement, others awaiting their call-up into the armed forces and refugees from the continent of Europe. They worked under difficult conditions. Many were killed and wounded. Many others were decorated, among them a little lady GP in the East End called Dr Hannah Billig, who was awarded both the George Medal and the MBE for heroism.

A few published papers on their experiences. Others gave vent to their feelings by contributing anonymously in the very popular column in the *Lancet*, which persists to this day, entitled 'In England Now'.

"In England now. A running commentary by peripatetic correspondents"

(1) *Lancet* 1941: i; 461–2

'The lights in the train suddenly went out and we knew that there was an air-raid in progress, but we ran on at a good pace in the bright moonlight, and I got to my home town only a little late. The station was in darkness, save for the shaded light belonging to the ticket collectors, and so we passed out into the streets to the noise of gunfire, the zoom of planes and the frequent crumps of bombs. There were no taxis, and I did not care at all for the prospect of walking the two or three miles home; so I decided to hurry along to my hospital, which was a good deal nearer, and give a hand in whatever was doing. I caught up with a soldier—an 'old sweat'—and we walked in step together. 'What a bloody party,' he said as a sudden brilliance lit up the sky, and we saw a 'Molotov chandelier' dropping down. 'That's so-and-so,' he went on, pointing to a huge fire behind us, 'Jerry knows where he bloody well is' (I found out later that it was nowhere near the important so-and-so).

Our ways parted and he clumped off into the moonlight, with a five-mile walk in front of him.

At hospital no casualties had yet come in, and my houseman took me to the residents' room for tea and toast. One of the other housemen came in from his shift of fire-watching, and we discussed where the fires in the town might be. Then came the news that a casualty had come in, and we trooped down to the reception hall. It was rather an anticlimax to find that he was an old man with a cerebral haemorrhage. But soon a real air-raid victim came in—a man who, standing at his door watching for incendiaries, had been thrown out into the street by the collapse of the house under a H.E. bomb. He had a fractured tibia and fibula, and he was covered with dust and dirt, his face as black as a coolie's. The next was a middle-aged Roman Catholic priest who, being unable to find a bag of sand in the street, had jumped on an incendiary bomb to put it out and had found it explode as he landed on it. Then came a couple of walking cases—bruised ribs from falling bricks, and a fire watcher whose tendo Achilles had been trodden on by a horse. He sat indignantly in a chair, nursing his sore heel and appealing to me. 'Why need the chap have interfered with the rope?' he said. 'What chap and what rope?' I asked. 'Well, when the bomb fell, I went to get the three horses out of the stable, and I'd got two out all right, and then this fellow comes along and grabs hold of the rope and mucks everything up. He'd no cause to get hold of the rope, I was managing nicely.' 'Were they your horses then?' I asked. 'No, they'd nothing to do with me, you know; but I knew they were there and had to be got out, and I was managing nicely. He'd no cause to get hold of the rope.' I looked at his foot, rather for form's sake, because as a physician I know a little about these things: obviously he was not badly hurt, only bruised and sore. 'Just like another famous chap,' I said. He looked at me quizzically; 'What famous chap?' 'A fellow called Achilles.' 'Never heard of him,' he said, with the generous air of letting me have my little joke, and an obvious relief that things were not beyond a joke.

An air-raid warden, white with dust, who had brought in the man with the fractured tibia, then tackled me. 'Eh doctor, d'you think there's any chance of my getting my best Sunday tie back again, it's round that first-aid splint? I expect I'll get a George Medal for tying up that leg! But I'd like that tie back again, I feel so untidy without a tie round my collar.' Even the fractured tib. and fib. on the stretcher ('Records' were just finishing his particulars) had to smile. Then came an elderly woman from the same incident, with great raw gaps of flesh torn out of her arm and leg, badly shocked, with a strange, uncanny look of puzzled questioning. Soon more cases were coming in, and I went along to the resuscitation ward. Already the tib. and fib., the priest and the elderly woman were being got into bed and warmed up. More cases arrived in the ward. There was an oldish man with a head wound, his clothes wringing wet, profoundly shocked, dazed and shivering. I never found out why he was soaked, and he could not tell me; but when I gave a hand with the surprisingly awkward task of taking off his wet and clinging trousers, he roused up and said angrily, 'Here, what are you doing that for?' Two policemen out of a posse of four who had been sent out to clear the streets round an unexploded bomb were carried in, nearly dead, with the skin blasted from their faces. One of our policemen had been blown a distance of fifty yards or more, and three days later they were still finding in the mass of rubble pieces of uniform and limbs belonging to the other two, as well as the bodies of other poor folk who had been buried. Happily our two constables still survive.

A middle-aged warden carried in a bundle, telling us that it was an unidentified child rescued from what had been a group of modern tenement dwellings. It was a little boy about a year old, his face waxen where it was not black with grime, with a pulpy wound on the back of the head, and a great gash across the forehead. For several hours we watched the baby's life ebb, and then slowly come back again with the appropriate resuscitation measures. An auxiliary fireman came with one of his mates, who had a deep wound in the knee-joint. They had been fighting one of the big fires in the town, playing their hoses from an adjoining building. An H.E. bomb hit their building, and my informant found himself standing on a beam high in mid-air.

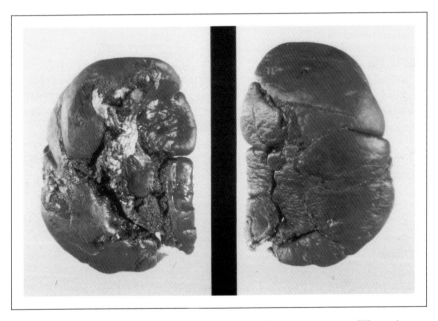

A sad memento from the blitzkrieg from the Museum at Westminster Hospital. The author often taught on this specimen. The catalogue reads: 'The spleen of a child aged two who received a fatal injury when a building collapsed during an air raid in October 1940. The spleen is ruptured in many places and the abdomen was full of blood at autopsy. No obvious bruising of the side was noted on admission but the child died soon afterwards'

He grabbed at his pal and held him for a second or two; when the man slipped out of his grasp. He fell on the debris of brick and building and not underneath it, and this saved his life, for three or four other A.F.S. men were crushed to death on the spot. His friend turned to me with savagely clenched fist. 'Shooting's too good for That Man,' he said.

All this time confident young registrars and housemen, sisters and nurses were getting on with their various jobs, and the emergency theatre was now in action. The tib.-and-fib., the priest, the elderly woman and others were back in bed, recovering from their anaesthetics. I was in the anteroom of the theatre, having a cigarette with my houseman, when suddenly there was a heavy explosion. My houseman dived under the theatre trolley, and rather like a slow-motion picture I dropped on to the floor on my face, listening to what sounded like the roof falling in, and foolishly aware that after all I had not even the cover of the thin aluminium top of the trolley. Then we got up again, and looked around the hospital to see where it had been hit. But it had not been hit; a very heavy bomb had landed on a building across the way. I rushed up to my own wards; glass and dust were all about the corridors, all the windows of one of my wards were broken and some in the other, but the patients were all safe. The night nurses had the situation in hand, the patients were steady and some could even crack a grim joke

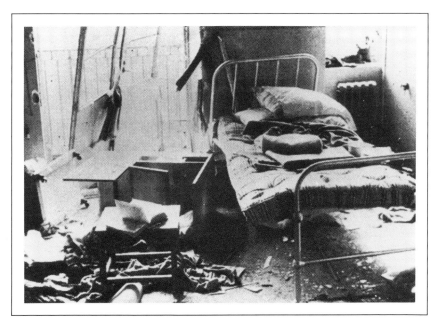

Annie Zunz Ward, Westminster Hospital. Damage produced by parachute mine on the night of 16 November 1940
(J. G. Humble and P. Hansell *Westminster Hospital* London: Pitman Medical, 2nd Edition 1974)

about it. It was the same throughout the hospital—glass and dust and soot, no casualties and no panic.

I went back again to the resuscitation ward, which was nearly full. We got some more beds in, and admitted more. The baby with the head wounds did not seem to be rallying. A woman who had been sitting in front of her kitchen fire had been badly burnt on the face, legs and abdomen when the blast of a bomb blew the fire out into the room. A young man, bending over the kettle to make some tea for his old mother had suffered a fracture of the spine when the roof fell in on him. A strapping young soldier, caught in the middle of the town when the raid began, was brought in unconscious after being hit by falling masonry. An old woman had several ribs cracked and a nasty shoulder wound; she died soon afterwards. There were more children, crushed under falling houses. Two old people who were still alive when put into the ambulance were dead when it reached hospital. A couple of young Roman Catholic priests came in and flitted about the ward, doing their offices for the gravely injured and comforting the others of their flock. I came to the bedside of a white-faced motionless young woman, and felt her pulse. On the other side of the ward the baby with the head wounds started to whimper protestingly under the electric warming cradle—rather a hopeful sound to the professional ear. The young woman opened her eyes and said 'Is my baby very badly hurt?' 'He's got a nasty gash or two,' I replied, 'but I think he's going to be all right.' A ghost of a smile passed over her face and was gone, and she closed her eyes again. It was her baby, and she too had been dug out of the debris, badly crushed, an hour or two after the child. She still survives, but her baby died thirty hours later.

My colleague the honorary surgeon had arrived, and we went round the beds together, weaving our way in and out of the stretchers which with the occupants were now filling up a large part of the floor. Such cases as were fit for operation in the course of the next hour or two could well be left to the younger men, so we made a tour of the wards. As we were doing this the all-clear went, so we could use our torches a little more freely. The moonlight was streaming in through gaps which had once been windows, making odd glinting patterns on the floors of the wards. Outside it was a lovely night, and some imp of memory flashed on the screen of my mind that scene of Lorenzo and Jessica's love-making:

Sit, Jessica, Look how the floor of heaven
Is thick inlaid with patines of bright gold;
There's not the smallest orb which thou behold'st
But in his motion like an angel sings,
Still quiring to the young-ey'd cherubims:
Still harmony is in immortal souls;
But whilst this muffy vesture of decay
Doth grossly close it in, we cannot hear it.

We took a provisional decision on the extent to which the hospital could continue to function, and gave our instructions for the coming day's evacuation of a large proportion of our patients to hospitals elsewhere. Downstairs the work went on, and would go on well into the afternoon, before the resuscitation ward could be cleared and tidied up and made ready again for the hazards of the next night. There was nothing more for us to do at the moment, and two of the ward sisters who were making a brew of tea called us in to share it. They had both got up and had been busy settling their own patients to sleep in the little corridors leading to the wards, and now all was quiet. We sat over sister's fire and chatted. The blitz had already fallen into its place and proportion in the life of our hospital; for our recollections of the night were not only of torn and crushed bodies, of shattered wards and narrow escapes, but also of old Daddy P., who somewhere about 3 am was found putting his thin legs out of bed. 'Here, Dad, where do you think you're going?' One of our party had said to him. The thin legs were slowly withdrawn again under the bedclothes. 'I'm sorry,' was the sleepy reply. 'I thought it was time to get up.'

(2) *Lancet* 1942: **ii**: 522–3

Among casualties admitted to a south Coast hospital during a recent air-raid was a man with an injured thigh. There was what looked like a wound of entry beneath which a sharp-pointed object could be felt. When the injury occurred the raiders had dropped all their bombs on a neighbouring town and were speeding home with their guns blazing. The object therefore was not a bomb fragment and was thought probably to be part of the fractured femur. X-rays however disclosed an unexploded aeroplane-cannon shell 8 by 2 cm., with its blunt end lying deeply and the apex tapering to a sharp point. The wound was dressed and the limb splinted. The Bomb Disposal Unit was consulted and the officer in charge visited the hospital and saw the radiograms. The shell he identified as of the armour-piercing variety which explodes on impact, and there were dark hints of a subvariety whose explosion is delayed. Removal was an obvious necessity, danger or no danger. Naturally the patient was left in blissful ignorance. The others in full knowledge of the facts got to work without fuss.

Within half an hour of leaving the ward the patient was back in bed. As the Chairman said days later at the hospital's annual bazaar, 'safely and successfully our surgeon had performed the most delicate and the most dangerous operation of his career.' When the operation was nearing completion the face of the assistant surgeon was seen at the theatre door. Asked what the dickens he wanted he replied, 'Only to know what my prospects are of promotion to the senior post.' The Chairman informed his audience that the ethics of his profession forbade him to disclose the surgeon's name. Subsequently, having incorrectly been himself designated in the press a surgeon, he has received embarrassing congratulations on his courage and skill, and his surpassing modesty in not disclosing his own name.'

Glossary and Abbreviations

AFS—Auxilary Fire Service
Blitz—(Blitzkreig), 'Lightning War', but commonly used slang for an air raid
HE—High Explosive
Molotov Chandelier—Cluster of incendiary bombs
'That Man'—Adolf Hitler

Reference

In England Now. A running commentary by peripatetic correspondents. *Lancet* 1941: **1**; 461–2; *Lancet* 1942: **ii**; 522–3.

Part III
Surgical Emergencies and Disasters

[21]

William Cheselden

1—Traumatic avulsion of the forequarter
2—Rupture of a strangulated umbilical hernia
(1778)

When I was a senior registrar in Oxford, I published my first book, which was on clinical anatomy. I was determined to produce a text that was readable and relevant to the student's needs. (I am glad to say that, 30 years later it is still going strong). One of the inspirations for this came to me when I purchased a copy of Edition 11 of William Cheselden's *The Anatomy of the Human Body,* first published in 1713 when he was a youth of 25. This small book maintained its popularity among students for more than a century, edition 13 appearing in 1792. Curiously enough, after the publication of its last edition in London, it began to have separate editions in America, the first appearing in 1795 and the second (which I

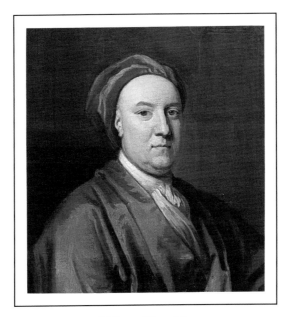

William Cheselden
(Reproduced by permission of the President and
Council of the Royal College of Surgeons of England)

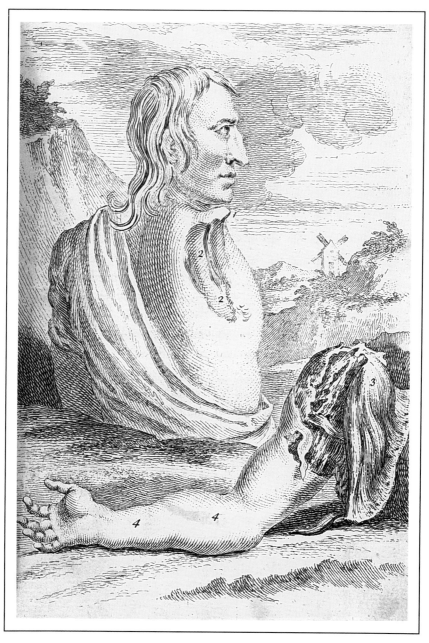

Traumatic forequarter avulsion—Samuel Wood.
(Cheselden *The Anatomy of the Human Body* London, 1778)

also possess) in 1806. The reason for its popularity was that it contained the essentials of gross anatomy mingled with physiological and clinical discussions.

Of the fascinating case reports therein, I have chosen two examples: one of a traumatic amputation of the shoulder, whose physiological lesson is as true today as in the eighteenth century; another of a strangulated umbilical hernia in an old lady. She recovered, but only at the expense of a permanent faecal fistula.

William Cheselden (1688–1752) was undoubtedly the foremost surgeon of his day in London. He was a pioneer of ophthalmic surgery, a master at cutting for the bladder stone, and the first surgeon in the United Kingdom who insisted on the importance of a sound knowledge of anatomy for the medical student and upon dissection to obtain this. A surgeon at both St Thomas's and Westminster Hospitals, he gave up these positions to devote himself entirely as surgeon to the Royal Hospital Chelsea, which had been founded by King Charles II for the care of old and disabled soldier pensioners. Today, he lies buried in its grounds. It was my great privilege to serve for many years as surgeon to this hospital, in very distant line of descent from William Cheselden.

William Cheselden "The Anatomy of the Human Body"

(11th Edition, 1778)

'The figure of Samuel Wood, a miller, whose arm with the scapula was torn off from his body, by a rope winding round it, the other end being fastened to the coggs of a mill (Figure, p. 132). This happened in the year 1737. The vessels being thus stretched bled very little, the arteries and nerves were drawn out of the arm, the surgeon who was first called placed them within the wound, and dressed it superficially. The next day he was put under Mr Ferne's care, at St Thomas's Hospital, but he did not remove the dressings for some days: The patient had no severe symptoms, and the wound was cured by superficial dressings only, the natural skin being left almost sufficient to cover it; which should in all cases be done as much as may be: Above twenty years since I introduced the method of amputating, by first dividing the skin and membrana adiposa, lower than the place where the operation was to be finished, the advantages of which are now sufficiently known.

The case of Margaret White, the wife of John White, a pensioner in the Fishmongers almshouses at Newington in Surrey. In the fiftieth year of her age, she had a rupture at her navel, which continued till her seventy-third year, when, after a fit of the cholic, it mortified, and she being presently after taken with a vomiting, it burst. I went to her and found her in this condition, which about six and twenty inches and a half of the gut hanging out, mortified. I took away what was mortified, and left the end of the sound

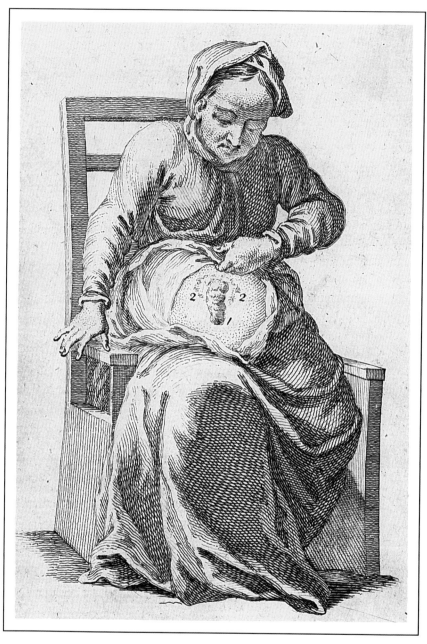

Intestinal fistula—Margaret White.
(Cheselden *The Anatomy of the Human Body* London, 1778)

gut hanging out at the navel, to which it afterwards adhered; she recovered, and lived many years after, voiding the excrements through the intestine at the navel; and though the ulcer was so large, after the mortification separated, that the breadth of two guts was seen; yet they never at any time protruded out at the wound, though she was taken out of her bed, and sat up every day (Figure, p. 134).'

References

Cheselden W. *The Anatomy of the Human Body*. 11th Edition. London: Printed for JF and C Rivington *et al*, 1778.
Cope Z. *William Cheselden*. Edinburgh: Livingstone, 1953.

[22]
Astley Cooper
1—Ligation of
the abdominal aorta (1817)
2—Fatal haemorrhage following
haemorrhoidectomy (1825)

Astley Cooper was one of the fathers of modern vascular surgery. He pioneered ligation of the carotid artery for aneurysm, he devised the extraperitoneal approach to the external iliac artery for femoral aneurysm, and, although the case ended fatally, he was the first surgeon to ligate the

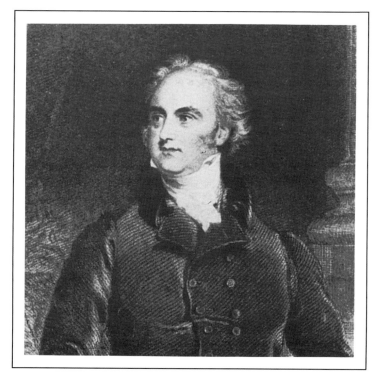

Sir Astley Paston Cooper
(Reproduced by permission of the President and Council of the Royal College of Surgeons of England)

abdominal aorta. This operation was performed in 1817 and it remained for Rudolph Matas, over a century later, to report the first successful ligation of the aorta for aneurysm in 1925.

Astley Cooper was born in 1768, the son of a Norfolk country clergyman. At the age of 16 he became articled to his uncle, William Cooper, who was the senior surgeon at Guy's Hospital. However, Astley lived with Henry Cline, surgeon at St Thomas's. In those days the two hospitals were opposite each other across St Thomas's Street, where Guy's remains to this day, and were known as the United Hospitals. Medical students were attached to both institutions, their lectures in medicine being at Guy's and those in surgery and anatomy at St Thomas's.

Cline encouraged young Cooper to attend the lectures of John Hunter and, six months after arriving in London, Astley transferred his apprenticeship to Cline. He now began his lifetime interest in anatomy. While still a pupil, he was appointed, first, demonstrator in anatomy and then, at the age of 23, helped Cline with his course of lectures.

Cooper was appointed to the surgical staff at Guy's Hospital in 1800 and there he spent the rest of his professional life.

He must have been one of the hardest working surgeons in history. At the height of his fame he would rise every morning by six, often by five and sometimes as early as four. He would go straight to his dissecting room, which was a shed in his own home, and there he would experiment until breakfast. From then until 1 o'clock he gave free consultations at his home. He then went to Guy's Hospital, where crowds of students would attend his ward rounds, clinical lectures and operating sessions. Visits to private patients and operations in their homes would follow. He would be home by seven, take a hurried meal, and then out again to see more patients or to lecture, rarely arriving home before midnight. He used to say that a day spent without dissection was a day wasted.

His enormous clinical practice made him one of the wealthiest surgeons of all time. For many years his income averaged £15,000 and in 1815 it reached the huge sum of £21,000; perhaps this should be multiplied by 100 to make it comparable with today's value. At one time his patients included King George IV, the Duke of York, the Prime Minister (Lord Liverpool) and the Minister of War (Lord Bathurst). In 1821 he removed a sebaceous cyst of the scalp from George IV, for which he was made a Baronet.

Cooper's contributions to surgery were considerable. In addition to his work on arterial ligation, he was one of the first surgeons to carry out a successful disarticulation of the hip. This procedure was performed in 1824 on a soldier wounded at the battle of Waterloo, with chronic osteomyelitis of the femur following an above knee amputation. His monograph on *Hernia*, published in 1804, gives an account of the anatomy of the groin which can be read with profit to this day. It contains the first description of the fascia transversalis, which he so named. His other monographs were

Dislocations and Fractures (1822), *Illustrations of Diseases of the Breast* (1829), *Observations on the Structure and Diseases of the Testis* (1830), *The Anatomy of the Thymus Gland* (1832) and *On the Anatomy of the Breast* (1840). The guiding principle in Cooper's teaching is stated in the preface to his treatise on *Hernia*, in which he states:

> 'I have almost uniformly in this work avoided quoting the opinion of authors on this part of surgery . . . I have therefore related no case, and given no remark to the truth of which I cannot vouch'.

At the age of 57, Astley Cooper resigned as Senior Surgeon to Guy's Hospital but continued with his private practice and his dissections. In 1827 he was elected President of the Royal College of Surgeons and in 1836 was elected for a second term in office. He died in 1841, at the age of 72, from what was probably hypertensive cardiac failure.

To return now to Cooper's contributions to vascular surgery. He was not simply a bold surgeon, who ligated most of the major arteries of the body, but his work was based on careful observation and experimental studies. While still a student, he investigated the collateral circulation in the dog following femoral and brachial artery ligation. He made extensive studies on ligation of the carotid and vertebral arteries and had one dog that actually survived serial ligation of all four of these vessels. In 1811 he reported successful ligation of the abdominal aorta in the dog and demonstrated specimens to demonstrate the collateral circulation which follows this. These specimens still survive in the museum at Guy's.

When, in 1817, a patient presented at Guy's Hospital with a rapidly expanding iliac aneurysm, which was obviously on the point of rupture, Cooper had the opportunity to put his experimental observations to test. At this point he went to the post mortem room and attempted to expose the aorta through a lateral retroperitoneal incision, found this to be 'utterly impracticable' and practised the trans-abdominal approach. His operation of aortic ligation had therefore been completely studied, both from its physiological and anatomical aspects.

As the following case report describes, the collateral circulation was indeed sufficient on the normal side, but on the side of the aneurysm, where collateral channels were no doubt disrupted and thrombosed, the leg became ischaemic and the patient died.

Oliver Cromwell once said to his artist 'paint me warts and all'. Astley Cooper was not a man to recount only his successes, and he did not hesitate to provide illustrative case histories of his disasters. The second case report shows that, in the early 19th century, even the highest in the land might face death from what, today, would be regarded as a fairly minor procedure of an operation for piles. Reading this second report makes one very grateful for the introduction of general anaesthesia and of the availability of blood transfusion!

Astley Cooper "Ligature on the aorta"

The lectures of Sir Astley Cooper, Bart. FRS Surgeon to the King etc etc on the Principles and Practice of Surgery Volume II London: Thomas and George Underwood, 69–72, 1825

'Charles Hutson, a porter, aet 38, was admitted into Guy's Hospital, on the 9th of April 1817, for an aneurysm in the left groin, situated partly above and partly below Poupart's ligament. The swelling was very much diffused, and pressure upon it gave considerable pain. On the third day after he had been in the Hospital, the swelling increased to double its former size, and extended for three to four inches above Poupart's ligament to an equal distance below it, and was of great magnitude. Just below the anterior and superior spinous process of the ilium, a distinct fluctuation could be felt in the aneurismal sac, so that the blood had not evidently yet coagulated; and the peritoneum was carried far from the lower part of the abdomen, in such a manner as to reach the common iliac artery, and to render an operation impracticable without opening the cavity of the peritoneum. I therefore was extremely averse to perform an operation, and determined to wait and see if any efforts would be made towards a spontaneous cure.

He was occasionally bled, kept perfectly quiet, and pressure was applied on the tumour. June 19th, a slough was observed on the exterior part of the swelling below Poupart's ligament, which, in part, separated on the 20th, and he had some bleeding from the sac, but it was easily stopped by a compress of lint, confined on the part by adhesive plaster. On the 22nd, after some slight exertion, he bled again, but not profusely. 24th, the bleeding again recurred, but stopped spontaneously. 25th, about half-past two o'clock, in consequence of a sudden mental agitation, bled profusely, and became so much exhausted, that his faeces passed off involuntarily; but Mr Key, then my apprentice, succeeded in preventing immediate dissolution by pressure. At nine o'clock the same evening I saw him, and found him in so reduced a state, that he could not survive another haemorrhage, with which he was every moment threatened. Yet still anxious to avoid opening the abdomen, to secure the aorta near to its bifurcation, I made an incision into the aneurismal sac, above Poupart's ligament, to ascertain if it were practicable to pass a ligature around the artery from thence. On introducing my finger, I found that the artery entered the sac above and quitted it below, without there being an intervening portion of vessel; I, therefore, was obliged to abandon that mode of operating; and as the only chance which remained of preventing his immediate dissolution, by haemorrhage, was by tying the aorta, I determined on doing it. The operation was performed as follows:

The patient's shoulders were slightly elevated by pillows, in order to relax, as much as possible, the abdominal muscles; for I expected that a protrusion of intestines would produce embarrassment in the operation, and was gratified to find that this was prevented by their empty state, in consequence of the involuntary evacuation of the faeces. I then made an incision, three inches long, into the linea alba, giving it a slight curve, to avoid the umbilicus: one inch and a half was above, and the remainder below the navel. Having divided the linea alba, I made a small aperture into the peritoneum, and introduced my finger into the abdomen; and then with a probe-pointed bistoury enlarged the opening into the peritoneum to nearly the same extent as that of the external wound. During the progress of the operation, only one small convolution of intestine projected beyond the wound.

Having made a sufficient opening to admit my finger into the abdomen, I passed it between the intestines to the spine, and felt the aorta greatly enlarged, and beating with excessive force. By means of my finger nail, I scratched through the peritoneum on the left side of the aorta, and then gradually passed my finger between the aorta and spine, and again penetrated the peritoneum, on the right side of the aorta.

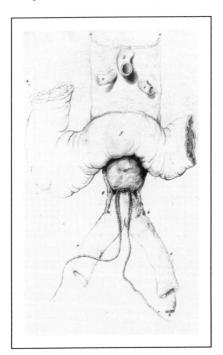 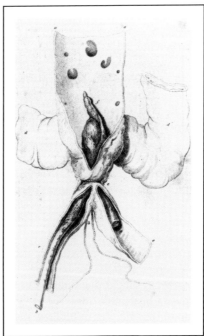

(A) Anterior View   (B) Posterior View
Contemporary drawings of Sir Astley Cooper's specimen of ligation of the abdominal aorta.
(Reprinted with permission from Guy's Hospital Reports 1940–1941. United Medical and Dental Schools, London)

I had now my finger under the artery, and by its side I conveyed the blunt aneurismal needle, armed with a single ligature behind it; and Mr Key drew the ligature from the eye of the needle to the external wound, when the needle was withdrawn.

The next circumstance, which required considerable care, was the exclusion of the intestine from the ligature, the ends of which were brought together at the wound, and the finger was carried down between them, so as to remove every portion of the intestine from between the threads: the ligature was then tied, and its ends were left hanging out of the wound.

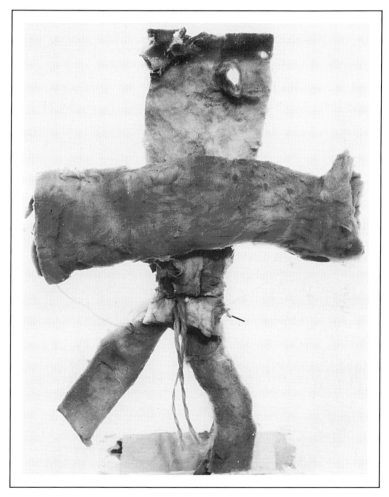

The specimen of Sir Astley Cooper's ligation of the abdominal aorta, preserved in the Department of Surgery at St Thomas's Hospital, London.

(Courtesy of Professor Norman Browse, PRCS)

During the operation the faeces passed involuntarily, and the patient's pulse, both immediately and for an hour after the operation, was 144 in a minute. I applied my hand to his right thigh, immediately after the operation, and he said that I touched his foot, so that the sensibility of the leg was very imperfect.

The omentum was drawn behind the opening as far as the ligature would admit, so as to facilitate adhesion; and the edges of the wound were brought together by means of a quilted suture and adhesive plaster.

He remained very comfortable until the following evening, when he vomited, and his faeces passed off involuntarily. 27th, Seven o'clock am, had passed a restless night, and had vomited at intervals; pulse 104, weak and small; pain in head; great anxiety of countenance; very restless, and his urine dribbled from him. He gradually sunk, and died at eighteen minutes after one o'clock, having survived the operation forty hours.

Dissection

No peritoneal inflammation, but at the edges of the wound, which were glued together by adhesive matter, excepting at the part at which the ligature protruded. The thread had been passed around the aorta, about three quarters of an inch above its bifurcation, and rather more than an inch below the part at which the duodenum crosses the artery; it had not included any portion of omentum, or intestine. Upon carefully cutting open the aorta, a clot, of more than an inch in length, was found to have sealed the vessel above the ligature; below the bifurcation, another, an inch in extent, occupied the right iliac artery; and the left was closed by a third, which reached as far as the aneurism: all were gratified to observe the artery so completely shut in forty hours. The aneurismal sac, which was of a most enormous size, reached from the common iliac artery to below Poupart's ligament, and extended to the outer part of the thigh. The artery was deficient from the upper to the lower part of the sac, which was filled with an immense quantity of coagulum.

"Fatal Haemorrhage following Haemorrhoidectomy"

Ibid pages 343–345

The Earl of S . . . applied to me for piles with prolapsus ani, and I removed some of the largest with scissars [sic]; the prolapsus was greatly relieved; and for more than 12 months after he was little troubled, either with haemorrhoids or prolapsus. About two years afterwards he again applied to me for a return of his complaint; and seeing his age, and having examined the piles, I thought before I operated, I would have a consultation, when the operation of excision was again recommended. I removed with the scissars one of the largest, and desired his Lordship to keep the recumbent posture. He laid down upon the bed immediately after the pile was removed. In about

10 minutes he said, 'I must relieve my bowels,' and he rose from his bed and discharged into the close stool what he thought to be faeces, but which proved to be blood. In 20 minutes he had the same sensation, and evacuated more blood than before, in about the same lapse of time; he again rose, and soon became very faint from the free haemorrhage. I, therefore, opened the rectum with a speculum, and saw an artery throwing out its blood with freedom, I therefore requested him to force down the intestine as much as he could, and raising the orifice of the bleeding vessel with a tenaculum, secured it in a ligature, and also compressed the artery with a piece of sponge. His Lordship bled no more. On the following day he was low, his pulse very quick, and he had a shivering: on the next day he complained of pain in his abdomen; he had sickness and tenderness upon pressure and in 4 days he died. In the presence of Mr Wardrop I opened his body, and found inflammation of the rectum, and disease of the glandulae solitariae of the intestine, they being enlarged and hardened, so that the intestine internally had a curious spotted appearance. He was not, therefore, a healthy or sound man in other respects; and it is in such cases that unexpected symptoms arise after operation.

As a ligation prevents the danger of bleeding, it is best to use it, although the process is more tedious and painful. The pain which it produces may be mitigated by not drawing the ligature too tight. Draw down the pile with forceps, or a tenaculum, and tie a piece of waxed silk around it, draw the knot until the patient complains severely, then tie a second, cut off the ligature a little way from the knot and return the intestine and pile.'

References

Brock RC. *The Life and Work of Astley Cooper.* Edinburgh: Livingstone, 1952.
Cooper A. *The Lectures of Sir Astley Cooper Bart FRS, Surgeon to the King etc etc on the Principles and Practice of Surgery; with additional notes on cases by Frederick Tyrell Esq.* Vol II (Case 1 pages 67–72, Case 2 pages 343–345) London: Thomas and George Underwood, 1825.

[23]
Sir Charles Bell
Haemorrhage from a cut throat (1828)

Sir Charles Bell was the prototype academic surgeon; not only a surgeon but also an anatomist, neurologist, experimental physiologist and artist. Like a true academic, he died a poor man and his widow had to receive a government pension to save her from living in penury.

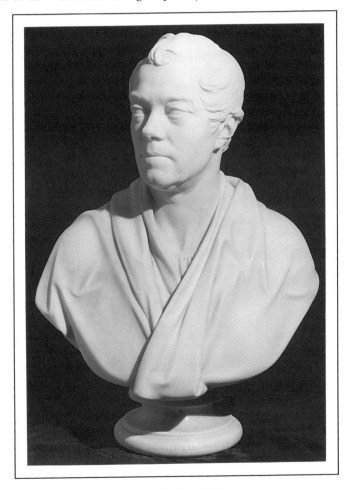

Sir Charles Bell
(Marble bust, Royal College of Surgeons of England. Reproduced by permission of the President and Council.)

Bell was born in Edinburgh in 1774. Both his father and grandfather were clergymen and his mother, his father's second wife, also had a clergyman father. Bell's elder brother, John, eleven years his senior, was an outstanding surgeon in Edinburgh at the close of the 18th Century and trained Charles in both Anatomy and Surgery. Not only did Charles assist his brother in his Anatomy School, but he also attended the University of Edinburgh, where the famous Professor Monro lectured in Anatomy. This Monro, nicknamed Monro Secundus, was the second of three generations of Monros, primus, secundus and tertius, that occupied the Chair of Anatomy for a consecutive period of 126 years. Secundus, the most distinguished of the three, occupied this important position for no less than half a Century.

Whilst still a student, Charles Bell published *A System of Dissection* in 1799, with plates engraved after his own drawings. This was followed in 1801, by his *Engravings of the Arteries and Nerves of the Brain.* These two works established his reputation at an early age as both an anatomist and an artist.

In 1804, at the age of 30, Charles left Edinburgh for London, where he taught anatomy, practised surgery and completed his *Essays on the Anatomy of Expression in Painting.* In 1812 he purchased the famous Great Windmill Street School of Anatomy, which had been founded by William Hunter, (elder brother of John), and which attracted students from all over the metropolis. Visitors to London today will find the site of this historic building to be the Lyric Theatre, and perhaps appropriately, the stage door marks the position of the old entrance through which cadavers were taken into the school!

Bell's appointment to the staff of the Middlesex Hospital in 1814, plunged him into a heavy load of surgical work and his reputation as a practical surgeon was extremely high, enhanced by his numerous and beautifully illustrated publications. These included *A System of Operative Surgery Founded on the Basis of Anatomy* and his *Illustrations of the Great Operations of Surgery, Trepan, Hernia, Amputation, Aneurysm and Lithotomy.*

The Battle of Waterloo took place on Sunday 18th June 1815. News of the battle took four days to reach London. Bell's response was immediate. Turning to his brother-in-law and fellow surgeon, John Shaw, he said 'Johnnie, how can we let this pass' and the two of them set off for Brussels, their only passports being their surgical instruments. They arrived at Waterloo eleven days after the battle and found many of the casualties, especially among the French, still unattended. For the first three days he operated day and night for spells of twelve or thirteen hours without a break and probably attended some 300 wounded. He continued, even under this stress, with the habit of a lifetime, making copious notes of his cases and sketches from which he later prepared the magnificent paintings, which can be seen to this day, for example, in the Museum of the Royal College of Surgeons of Edinburgh. He also brought back many specimens, still to be seen, illustrating gun-shot wounds from the Waterloo campaign.

Bell's reputation as a scientist today rests on his studies of the nervous system. He demonstrated, in animal experiments on the exposed spinal cord, that pricking or injuring the posterior nerve roots produced no muscle contraction whereas injury to the anterior filaments resulted in muscle convulsion. These experiments were extended by Magendie in Paris in 1822, who demonstrated that division of the posterior nerve roots in puppies abolished sensation but allowed limb movement to persist. Magendie was then able to carry out the difficult procedure of dividing the anterior roots while preserving the posterior nerves and recorded abolition of movement but not of sensation. This demonstration of the functions of the anterior and posterior nerve roots has come to be termed the Bell-Magendie rule. Bell also performed detailed experimental studies in the ass of the trigeminal and facial nerves and demonstrated the predominantly sensory function of the former and entirely motor action of the latter. Neurological cases came to Bell from all over the country and his description of idiopathic facial paralysis retains the eponym of Bell's palsy to this day. This syndrome he described in the Philosophical Transactions of the Royal Society in 1821. Ten years later he was knighted.

In 1836 Bell accepted the invitation to return to Edinburgh as Professor of Surgery at a salary of £400 a year. Shortly afterwards, he developed increasingly severe angina and died in 1842.

During his life, Charles Bell had an enormous reputation as a teacher. This case report, which comes from one of his clinical lectures recorded in the London Medical Gazette, gives some idea of the impact which his words must have had on his students, as well as giving us a flavour of the life of a surgeon in the early part of the 19th Century.

Charles Bell "Observations of Haemorrhage"

The London Medical Gazette 1828, Volume 1. Number 13, 361–365

'The peculiar excellence of Clinical instruction is owing to the state of preparation of the student's mind to receive an impression.

Sitting here you do not feel that I am speaking to you of things that may occur, by some remote chance, years hence, in your own practice, but on the contrary you see my anxiety, and partake of it. I particularly allude to the subject of haemorrhage: you have today seen the bleeding returning after amputation, notwithstanding every precaution: and yesterday, before you had left the hospital, you found I was called back to tie the femoral artery, owing to a secondary haemorrhage taking place after the operation for aneurysm.

As the accident occurred during the visit, you must all have partaken, in some measure, of the panic of the attendants, and the agitation of the patient, whose fate was impending whilst a pupil compressed the artery at the groin. You are prepared to understand the truth of the observation, that a surgeon to be expert and active, must previously, with deliberation, have studied the principles which are to guide him in these operations. Boldness, bodily activity, and even a knowledge of anatomy, will not avail him on such occasions unless he be directed by correct principles . . .

I myself may describe to you a scene which has just happened: it tends at least to remind you how unexpectedly we may be called upon to act.

I was coming home late at night, or rather when it was morning, the streets deserted, and the gas lights seeming to shine for the exclusive enjoyment of watchmen and women of the town. What occurred to me might well have suggested the description given by Defoe of London in the time of the plague when, as he went through the desolate streets, he heard a woman who had lost all her children, calling from her window 'Death, Death!'. As I turned round into one of the squares, a window was suddenly raised, and a lady screamed out 'My husband has cut his throat and is bleeding to death, will nobody bring a surgeon?' You will allow it was singular that at such a time there was a hospital surgeon passing beneath her window. I rushed into the house, but was admitted with some difficulty; the people of the house being alarmed, and naturally afraid of admitting improper persons. I made my way to the drawing-room and here I was met with a new obstacle; for the lady when she saw me and knew who I was, embraced me closely, beseeching my assistance, yet holding me so that I could not move. At last I threw her from me and going into the bedroom found her husband lying on his back, the blood streaming from his neck. I immediately caught hold of the vessel in the angle of the wound. After having secured it between my finger and thumb, I looked round for further assistance. Instead of finding my usual assistant, (my friend here, the house surgeon, to whose attention we are so much indebted), I was somewhat puzzled when I saw one who had on a large, shaggy, white great coat; an old hat, with broad brim upon his head and a red night cap under it, a beard of a fortnight's growth, and a chequered shawl around his neck. 'Sir' he said, 'I am off my beat, I hope you will have the kindness to answer for me why I have left it'.

I found that it was the watchman who was my assistant, he had followed me upstairs without my noticing him. I satisfied the old man that I would readily explain for him the occasion of his being off his beat. I was obliged to wait for some time, holding the bleeding vessels between my fingers, until some medical assistants arrived with ligatures and needles. I was much relieved when an old house surgeon of this hospital, Mr Tuson, made his appearance, with proper apparatus; and to him I resigned the care of the patient. The arteries were tied, the wound was then sewed, and properly done up.

It is thus, that having once entered upon the study of our profession, no matter what may be your intentions about practising only some particular branch of it, it is incumbent upon you to study everything relating to haemorrhage. Being a medical man, if an accident required sudden and prompt assistance, and you happen to be near, all the bystanders turn to you, and call upon you to afford the necessary aid. I may here repeat that there can be not true presence of mind unless you have studied with care the most essential of all subjects—the surgery of the arteries.'

References

Bell C. Observations on haemorrhage. *London Medical Gazette* 1828; **Vol 1,** No 13: 361–5

Gordon-Taylor G, Walls EW. *Sir Charles Bell, His Life and Times.* Edinburgh: Livingstone, 1958.

[24]

John Howship

Ruptured aortic aneurysm: strangulated umbilical hernia (1840)

A pleasant relaxation for any surgeon, from the most junior resident to the Chief of surgery, is to browse through some of the great old surgical text books. Those of the first half of the ninteenth century, which are not difficult to find in hospital libraries, are particularly readable. Surgical giants like Astley Cooper and John Hilton recount their failures and their successes in almost equal proportions, written in a style now long lost and replaced,

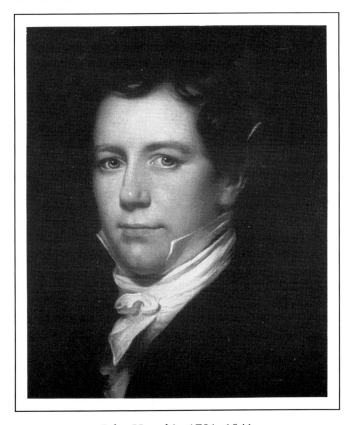

John Howship 1781–1841
(Reproduced by permission of the President and Council of the
Royal College of Surgeons of England.)

unfortunately, by the stacatto standard idiom of today's reportage, where "the patient died" is now translated as "the patient underwent negative care outcome".

A good example is John Howship's *Practical Remarks on the Discrimination and Appearances of Surgical Disease* published by John Churchill of London in 1840. From this I shall quote two extracts; the sad and inevitably fatal (in those days) progression of a thoracic aortic aneurysm, and successful operation, (without, of course, the benefits of anaesthesia), on a strangulated umbilical hernia.

John Howship was born in 1781. After serving as a surgeon in the army he was appointed assistant surgeon at Charing Cross Hospital in 1834 and became full surgeon two years later. He was a Member of the Royal College of Surgeons, (the Fellowship was only introduced in the Charter of 1843), and served on its Council. He was widely known in his time and was a member of medical societies in Paris, Dresden, Bonn and Copenhagen, as well as being a member of the Faculty of Medicine and Surgery of New Brunswick.

He wrote a large number of text books which included *Practical Observations in Surgery and Morbid Anatomy* and *Practical Observations on the Diseases that Affect the Secretion and Excretion of Urine.*

Unusual for a surgeon of his times, he was an expert in the use of the microscope. His name is preserved eponymously to this day in the term 'The Lacunae of Howship', the microscopic cellular spaces in bone. His interest in bone might be put down to the fact that he himself suffered from chronic osteomyelitis of the tibia, which caused him to walk with a pronounced limp.

He was a man of private means and lived comfortably in a house in Saville Row.

He died in 1841 'after a dangerous illness and several operations'.

John Howship "Practical remarks on the discrimination and appearances of surgical diseases"

London: Churchill, 1840

'Aneurysm of the Ascending Aorta, protruding through the Ribs into the Breast

S. B., 37, under care of Mr Houlton, had nine years previously received a severe blow on the left upper ribs, by the fall of a bedstead, and soon after felt internal pains, shooting, and throbbing, and within twelve months a pulsating tumour, the size of a hen's egg, projected through the ribs, with dreadful pains between the shoulders. Her treatment, occasional bleedings and low diet, had been her main dependence ever since; the swelling and pulsation gradually increased, stormy and windy weather always exciting increased violence and acute pain, darting through the shoulders and down the left arm.

Soon after I first saw the case, a small soft painless swelling appeared over the cartilage of the fourth left rib. The skin became thin; in coughing it broke, and by a minute opening discharged a teacupful of blood and serum, without relief to her internal feelings.

Calling one day, groaning with intense pain, she was immediately relieved by bleeding. On enquiry, the cause proved the strong susceptibility of this disease to be acted upon by moral impressions. A kind woman who administered liberally to her temporal wants, desirous to afford her spiritual comfort also, requested a clergyman to favour her with a call; the gentleman walked into her room, a total stranger, and without her suspecting who he was, or why sent; he said he could see she was very ill, enquiring abruptly what sort of life she had led? A question which probably elicited an offensive answer. Having, it seems, heard of some past moral delinquency in this poor woman's character, and thinking further preface unnecessary, instead of admonishing her with gentleness, he told her at once that she was in the high road to hell, and would soon be there. The resentment and rage thus excited was such, that on calling in, an hour or two after, I found the circulation excessively disturbed, and her sufferings and moans dreadful, while all she could say was expressive of regret that she had not had the strength enough to drive him out of the house, for conduct so inhuman.

The outward swelling occupied the left breast, which was much larger than the right, the glandular structure appearing to be partially removed by absorption. The swelling, she observed, was twice as large in winter as in summer, the pulsation then more powerful, and breathing more difficult. At the wrist, the left pulse was weakest and smallest.

She distinguished two kinds of pain, one at the heart, always relieved by bleeding, the other dispersed about the swelling and chest, extending to the side and shoulder, never relieved by bleeding. Three weeks before death, she felt something crack in the tumour, and the breast presently swelled to four or five times its previous bulk, becoming tense and livid. A little opening then formed in the skin, and another similar to it, on the other side of the breast, occasionally discharged blood and serum, and this discharge suddenly increasing, the pulse quickened, the strength sunk, and in a few days she died.

Post Mortem

On opening the chest we found the dilatation had commenced just above the origin of the aorta, and the whole of the ascending portion and curvature were much expanded, the anterior part forming a tumour larger than an orange, closely attached to the five upper ribs, by a circle about six inches in diameter. The anterior parts, and cartilages of the second, third and fourth ribs partially absorbed, had afforded space for the increase of the tumour, externally. The dilated aorta laid open, its internal surface was observed to be diseased, and in parts ossified, but contained no laminated or fibrinous coagula. The sternum, divided longitudinally, and a small bit removed by the saw, opposite the disease, brought into view the extension of the sac from the chest, through the pectoral muscle, into the breast. The breast laid open, exposed the remains of the whitish flattened glandular mass, and a large quantity of dark grumous blood in the superficial cellular tissue, the consequence of the recent diffusion of the fluid contents of the aneurism beneath the skin.

Strangulated Umbilical Hernia—Operation—Two openings through the Linea Alba, and two Protusions into one Sac

Mrs B., a very stout woman, 50, under care of Mr Egleton, had for many years an umbilical hernia, which had been strangulated for three days.

This evening (Sunday) Mr E. had infused one drachm of tobacco in a pint of boiling water, an hour, and injected six ounces of the infusion, and was then enabled to reduce a bit of intestine from the tumour, which he felt gurgling as it went back; and now at its upper part the sac felt somewhat flaccid, as if partially empty, the finger perceiving the little opening into the abdomen. Yet the patient lay groaning and moaning, bad as ever, and saying she was dying. Pulse below 60. Abdomen very tender, tumour painful. Her husband, she said, had been pulling it about all day, and sent for Mr E. yesterday evening. No stool since Thursday, but frequently sickness and retching; she was bled and ordered aperients.

Monday, four p.m. I operated; dividing the skin and subjacent tissues with care soon exposed the omental contents of the sac, the opening into which I freely enlarged on a director, dividing several strong bands. At the upper part of the tumour, beneath the omentum, was a small bit of intestine, which, by the gentlest pressure, retired through the opening in the linea alba so readily, as to evince that it could scarcely have been the seat of strangulation. This led me to examine very carefully a small mass of compact omentum in the lower part of the tumour; when I soon felt a transverse ridge, and separating the portions of small intestine, protruded through a second opening in the linea alba into the same sac; the one opening about an inch below the other. Endeavouring to effect the reduction without dividing the stricture; the patient exclaiming 'it is going up'. When returned, I examined, and found that the lower opening, the largest, had given passage to the omentum, which was adherent, and consequently allowed to remain. The pain and sickness immediately subsiding, the parts were brought together and soon united. The bowels acted freely and frequently, and she soon recovered.'

References

Howship J. *Practical Remarks on the Discrimination and Appearances of Surgical Disease*. London: Churchill, 1840.
Minney RJ. *Charing Cross—The Story of a Famous Hospital*. London: Cassell, 1967.

[25]

Augustus Eves

Ligation of the common carotid artery (1849)

Cheltenham is a sleepy, peaceful, pleasant country town situated among the green fields and rolling farm lands of 'middle England'. Elderly retired senior army officers and their lady wives, in the days of the British Empire, would return from a life-time spent in the blazing heat of India or one of our far-flung colonies to settle there. Nothing very dramatic ever happens in Cheltenham.

In the early 19th Century, the local surgeon in Cheltenham was a Mr Augustus Eves. Born in 1799, he had taken the qualification of MRCS in 1821. When the Fellowship of the Royal College was

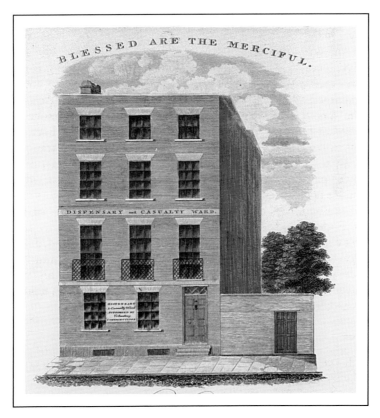

The Cheltenham Dispensary
(Courtesy of Maryse Roberts, Cheltenham postgraduate Medical Centre)

established, he was one of the many elected to the Fellowship without examination in 1844. He served for many years as surgeon to the Cheltenham General Hospital and supplemented his income by serving as referee to the Railway Passengers Assurance Company. He died on October 22nd 1868.

The one really exciting thing that happened to Augustus Eves took place on April 2nd 1847, an event he probably relived and retold many times until his dying day. It was then that he tied the common carotid artery of a man who had slit his throat in a suicidal attempt and who was moribund from haemorrhage. The case report, which he published in the Lancet two years later, makes fascinating reading.

Of course he was no pioneer in this operation. The credit for this goes to a British Naval Surgeon, David Fleming, who tied the common carotid artery in October 1803 for a secondary haemorrhage following a cut throat. This operation was carried out in the sick-bay of His Majesty's Ship 'Tennant', cruising off the Spanish coast. His patient, a ship's servant, had almost exsanguinated but made an uninterrupted recovery following his emergency operation (Keevil 1949).

Astley Cooper ligated the common carotid artery successfully at Guy's Hospital in 1808 in a man aged 50 for a massive carotid aneurysm at the bifurcation. A number of further cases, both for trauma and for aneurysm was subsequently reported in the first half of the nineteenth century—all, of course, carried out without the advantage of an anaesthetic. However, none of these would have disturbed the quiet life of a Cheltenham surgeon like the case described below:

A Eves Esq FRCS "Report of a case of suicidal wound of the throat with profuse haemorrhage successfully treated by ligature of the common carotid artery"

Lancet 1849; 1: 556

'On April 2nd, 1847, about eleven o'clock pm, I was sent for to a man named J, about forty-five years of age, living at the Knap, in this town. I found Dr Brookes, Mr Gregory and Mr Gregory, jun., in attendance on the patient, who was lying perfectly insensible and deluged with blood; the bedroom had the appearance of a slaughter-house rather than of a sleeping apartment. From Dr Brookes I learnt the following particulars; that he had found the patient with a wound extending from the angle of the jaw on the left side to within an inch of the same point on the right side; the larynx was not divided, nor was the cavity of the mouth penetrated. This wound was inflicted by the patient himself, by means of a sharp-pointed, curved pruning-knife. It was said that he stabbed himself three times with this instrument, apparently in the angle of the jaw on the left side, afterwards drawing the knife transversely across the throat.

The wound has been inflicted about half an hour before Dr Brookes saw the patient and was filled with a large coagulum, on removing which, to examine the nature of the injury, a gush of arterial blood, in a large stream, immediately poured forth from a great depth in that part of the wound situated in the angle of the jaw. Pressure was instantly applied and complete syncope came on, during the continuance of which the bleeding was greatly diminished and the wound was brought together by means of sutures, in the hope that the haemorrhage would not return. However, when reaction was again set up, the bleeding re-commenced as profusely as ever, until syncope again took place.

At this point I saw him, lying perfectly insensible, with the throat distended with an enormous coagulum and blood still gently flowing from the wound. I then cut the sutures, and turned out the coagulum but the man being very full about the neck the wound was so deep that we could not discover the bleeding vessels. The position of the patient, and the difficulty of throwing a strong light into the bottom of the wound were circumstances which also added to our perplexity. He was now lying in a state of insensibility, with occasional convulsive movements of different parts of the body and all present considered his case hopeless, and expected every moment to see him expire. His pulse at the wrist had quite ceased. Under these circumstances, I thought it would be giving him a slight chance of recovery, if the common carotid were tied below the omohyoideus muscle. This being agreed to, I cut down to the artery, guided by the inner edge of the sterno-cleido mastoideus muscle; the artery, when found, was perfectly flaccid and empty of course, without pulsation. The aneurysm needle was gently insinuated under it from the outside; the vessel was slightly raised, so that it could be ascertained that the nervus vagus was not on the needle; the ligature was then tied; and the wound made by the operation brought together by sutures. During the whole of this procedure the patient was perfectly insensible and manifested no feeling whatever. There was not any gush of blood after this, but a slight flow continued until we again brought the wound together by sutures, adhesive plaster and bandage. Before doing this we examined the wound and tied the two of three open mouths of vessels. In two or three hours the patient gradually began to rally and to my great surprise and satisfaction, when I visited him the next morning, I found reaction fully established. He had great difficulty in swallowing for some days; at first he only took a teaspoonful of milk occasionally through the day, whenever the person in charge could get him to attempt it. As we found the suicidal propensity still predominant, he was constantly watched with care and as soon as he was strong enough to be removed, which I think was about the tenth day after the perpetration of the rash act, I sent him to the Gloucester Lunatic Asylum. The wound in the throat healed by granulation and Dr Williams, the resident medical officer of the Gloucester Asylum, had the kindness to inform me that the ligature on the carotid came away on the 27th April being twenty-five days after the operation. He also mentioned the fact, which I afterwards had an opportunity of observing with him, that the muscles of the left side of the tongue were paralyzed, doubtless owing to injury of the ninth nerve, and evidenced by the point being invariably turned to the left side when protruded.

Considering the situation of the wound in this case, and the effects produced, I am almost led to believe that either the common carotid artery was wounded just before its bifurcation or one or both of the carotids immediately after its division; the superior thyroid was also doubtless divided; and perhaps the lingual and possible the facial, shared the same fate, as in some instances they are given off very closely together. . .

Since the above particulars were arranged, I have heard from Dr Williams of the death of J, which happened about fourteen months after the ligature of the carotid. The suicidal propensity continued very strong until nearly the end of his life; he died extremely emaciated, owing, in the opinion of Dr Williams, to disease of the mucous membrane of the stomach and bowels. Owing to a number of pressing engagements happening at the moment Dr Williams had not time to make a post-mortem examination.'

Note: Sadly no portrait of Augustus Eves can be found.

References

Eves A. Report of a case of suicidal wound of the throat with profuse haemorrhage, successfully treated by ligature of the common carotid artery. *Lancet* 1849; i: 556.
Keevil JJ. David Fleming and the operation for ligation of the carotid artery. *British Journal of Surgery* 1949; 37: 92–5.

[26]

H. C. Markham

Splenectomy for traumatic prolapse of the spleen (1874)

Just as the early history of intestinal surgery comprised the repair of prolapsed lacerated bowel, so the first authenticated cases of splenectomy, dating from the sixteenth century and well documented in the seventeenth century, were examples of the spleen, prolapsed and perhaps lacerated following a knife wound, being removed wholly or in part by a surgeon.

The first detailed account of survival after splenectomy for a prolapsed spleen resulting from trauma was given by Timothy Clark in 1676.

Already, in 1663, he had removed the spleen from a stray dog who lived for a year, put on flesh, 'became tamer than before, and was subsequently enthusiastic in its pursuit of sexual activity.' His account of his splenectomy in man, (translated from the Latin), reads:

'A butcher named William Panier, living in the village of Wayford, near Crookhome, in the County of Somerset, being greatly in debt, and fearing that lest he should be arrested, was constrained to go into hiding. The constables were about to capture him, and becoming desperate, and in order to avoid them, he drove his butcher's knife into his abdomen on the left side, thus causing a great wound through which part of the omentum, and of the intestine, and also the spleen protruded. The constables were horrified, and left the man for dead, as they believed. For three days the wound remained without a suture, but at last a surgeon was summoned. The surgeon replaced the intestines, and cut away part of the omentum, along with the spleen. The man rapidly recovered from the effects of the wound, and for the whole of the following year remained in good health and spirits. He soon afterward emigrated to New England, where not long ago he was so far living a healthy life.'

No details can be found of this truly remarkable English surgeon and experimentalist.

The second well-authenticated case of removal of the protruding spleen through a knife wound was performed by Nicolaus Matthias and was reported from Colberg in 1684.

Francis Home served as surgeon to a dragoon regiment in the War of Austrian Succession. He was present at the Battle of Dettingen in 1743. He reports in his *Medical Facts and Experiments*, published in London in 1759, the following interesting case:

'I was present at a very unusual operation in the morning after the Battle of Dettingen; when Mr Wilson, surgeon to Sir Robert Richards' dragoons, cut off most of the spleen from the dragoon. The wound being very large the spleen had come out, and being inflamed by the cold of the night, it could not be reduced. There was no possibility to get a formentation to apply to it. We therefore thought, that cutting it off was the only means to prevent mortification. The dragoon, although otherwise much wounded, recovered; and I saw him afterwards in good health. He had no stronger inclination for women than before.'

One should note carefully this early physiological observation on the effect of splenectomy!

American readers, in particular, will be especially fascinated with an account by Dr H. C. Markham of successful removal of traumatic prolapse of the spleen in an Indian patient, carried out under most difficult circumstances and with the aid of a medicine man and copious amounts of whiskey. In spite of some careful research, no further information can be found about this redoubtable surgeon.

H. C. Markham "Excision of a portion of the spleen—recovery"

Medical Record 1874; 9: 482-3

'The novel character of the following case, surgically and otherwise, may seem to give it a 'sensational' tinge: if so, the circumstances themselves are responsible, instead of any desire on the part of the writer to give it such an aspect.

At the instance of, and accompanied by the sheriff of the county, I visited an Indian of the Winnebago tribe, who in an altercation with a white desperado had received, as was supposed, fatal injuries. The object of my visit was to enable me to appear in court as a witness against the supposed murderer, more than to attempt any professional assistance. Arriving at the small Indian encampment, we found the object of our visit lying upon the ground in his wigwam, attended by a genuine 'Indian doctor'. Examination revealed no less than seven incised wounds upon the trunk and extremities; some of the wounds were six inches in length, but none had severed any important vessel. Owing to the peculiar and effective treatment of the 'medicine man', these wounds were doing well. Curiosity induced me to observe the method of treating these huge wounds, and so well was it repaid that it may be pardonable to describe it. The native surgeon obliged an aged squaw to carefully lick the surfaces of the cuts, after which—using his mouth as a syringe—he injected them with a wash of a dark color, the value of which the fine condition of the wounds well attested. Native skill, however, was baffled by one of the wounds, the principal feature of which induces this report. The wound penetrated the cavity of the abdomen, and was situated immediately over the region of the spleen. Through this wound the desperate struggles of the Indian with his enemy had forced the spleen to the extent of three-fourths its volume, the extreme projecting portion or border, from constriction at the wound and the extreme heat of the season, had already become sphacelated, about thirty-six hours having elapsed since the infliction of the wound. This wound, owing to its grave character, had been left to itself, the 'doctor' by grave signs confessing his inability to treat it. To enlarge the wound and return the organ in the condition then existing was out of the question, to leave it was, in my belief, equally unwarrantable—to remove it presented little better hope other than would arise from the scientific interest involved in the result. This interest impelled me to take charge of this 'section' of the case, being satisfied that the other wounds were in safe hands and did not seriously imperil life. After preparing ligatures, with a common bistoury the spleen was removed by making a section nearly on a plane with the surface of the abdomen. In spite of the constriction the haemorrhage was appalling, but with the assistance of my friend, the sheriff, I succeeded in applying ligatures sufficient to arrest it. The pulse was absent, and nothing but an early fatal issue seemed possible. Whiskey was given freely and cold water dressings used, with instructions to continue them. I saw no more of the case at that time, and was surprised some weeks after to learn that the party arrested for the killing had been released. About one year from the date of my medico-legal visit, an Indian came into my office smiling, and drawing aside his blanket, exhibited the cicatrix of a wound that was at once recognized. His only statement was 'Indian heap no run.' Accepting the usual theory of physiologists, and in view of the fact that his spleen was then in my possession, his laconic expression required no verification.

Although the entire organ was not removed it cannot be doubted that the portion remaining was wholly useless. The case determines the question as to the vital nature of the organ, and compels the admission that it throws much light upon an interesting physiological problem. A point of minor interest rests in the illustration it furnishes of the remarkable power of resistance to injury in this race, and contrasting with that of the 'pale face' whose habits of life are at such divergence with these children of nature.'

References

Ellis H. *The Spleen,* Austin: Silvergirl, 1988

Markham HC. Excision of a portion of the spleen—recovery. *Medical Record* 1874; 9: 482–3.

[27]
Charles McBurney
Early operative treatment of acute appendicitis (1889)

The first appendicectomy was performed by Claudius Amyand, surgeon to Westminster Hospital, London, in 1736. He operated on a boy, aged 11, who had a persistent faecal fistula in a right scrotal hernia. Within the scrotum he discovered the appendix perforated by a pin. The appendix was ligated and removed, with recovery.

Turning now to the development of the operative treatment of acute appendicitis, in 1864 Henry Hancock in London successfully drained an

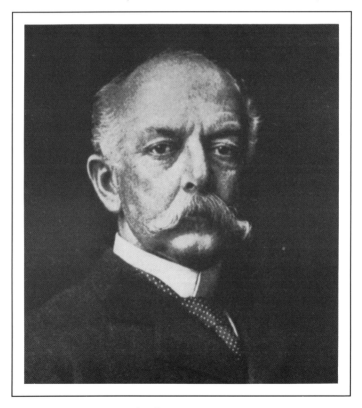

Charles McBurney
(Reproduced with permission from *American Journal of Surgery* February 1931)

appendix abcess in a 30 year old woman who was in her eighth month of pregnancy. William Parker of New York advised early incision in the treatment of appendix abcess in 1867. Following his report, many similar accounts were published.

In 1880, Lawson Tait of Birmingham operated on a patient with a gangrenous appendix. The patient recovered after removal of the offending organ. However, he did not report this case until 1890; therefore, credit for the first published account of 'appendicectomy' must go to Rudolf Kronlein, although the patient reported in 1886, a boy aged 17, died two days later. In 1887, T. G. Morton of Philadelphia correctly diagnosed and excised an acutely inflamed appendix lying within an abcess cavity. This was just one year after Reginald Fitz, professor of medicine at Harvard, gave a lucid and logical description of the clinical features of the condition as well as coining the term 'appendicitis'. Fitz was unusual as a professor of medicine in advocating early operation!

The challenge was taken up by Charles McBurney of New York, who pioneered early diagnosis and early operative intervention. He also devised the muscle-splitting incision named after him. He described 'McBurney's point' as the point of maximum tenderness in this condition.

Charles McBurney was born in 1845 in Roxbury, now a suburb of Boston. He was educated at Harvard and the College of Physicians and Surgeons, New York, qualifying in medicine and becoming a surgical intern at Bellevue Hospital at the age of 25. In 1875, he became attending surgeon at St Luke's and five years later became assistant surgeon at Bellevue. At the age of 43, he was given the entire surgical service of Roosevelt Hospital, a position he held for the succeeding 12 years, and served as professor of surgery at the College of Physicians and Surgeons.

In 1908 at the age of 63, he retired because of ill health and died aged 68, in 1913, of heart failure.

An important paper, from which this case report is quoted, began McBurney's advocacy of early intervention in acute appendicitis. For the following ten years, he published at least one paper anually on appendicitis. In this paper, the author also locates the point of maximum tenderness in appendicitis: 'very exactly between an inch and a half and two inches from the anterior spinous process of the ilium on a straight line drawn from that process to the umbilicus'.

Charles McBurney "Experience with early operative interference in cases of disease of the vermiform appendix"

New York Medical Journal 1889; 50: 676–684

'**Case 1**—EMP, a young gentleman nineteen years of age, complained of general abdominal pain at 11 am on May 21, 1888. The pain was regarded as due to indigestion, and was treated with family remedies. In the afternoon the patient fainted, and by four o'clock his pain had greatly increased in severity. He received a little morphine and hot applications were applied. At 5 pm his mouth temperature was 98.4°, his pulse 100. During the night and the following day the patient complained sometimes of severe pain, and occasionally felt much better; he took a considerable quantity of milk, and at 8 pm his temperature was only 100°. During the second night he suffered much pain, and at 5 am on the 23rd it was noted that his pain was chiefly in the right iliac fossa. At 5:30 he had a severe chill and his temperature rose to 103°, his pulse to 120. At this time he was visited by his physicians, Dr Fessenden N. Otis and Dr William K. Otis, who diagnosticated at once acute appendicitis, and requested me to see the patient. This I did at about 8:30. I found the pulse and temperature as stated, and the following condition: great rigidity of right abdominal muscles; exquisite tenderness on pressure at a point just two inches internal to the anterior spine of the ilium, in the direction of the umbilicus. Beneath the finger at this point could be felt a small resisting mass, less than one inch in diameter. No dullness on percussion anywhere. General appearance excellent. The diagnosis of appendicitis already made by Dr Otis was confirmed by myself, and an hour later by Dr Sands. Immediate operation advised and accepted. General appearance of patient excellent. It should be noted that at 11:30 the temperature had fallen to 101°.

Operation at 12 o'clock just forty-nine hours from the first pain. Present Dr F. N. Otis, Dr William K. Otis, Dr L. R. Morris, and Dr Tuttle.

Ether anaesthesia. A slightly oblique incision four inches and a half long, the center of this incision being two inches from the anterior iliac spine toward the umbilicus. Tissues of abdominal wall quite markedly edematous, particularly near the peritoneum. On opening the peritoneum freely, the appendix came at once into view. It was larger than a man's thumb, dark-brown in color, tense, evidently full of fluid, and at no point gangrenous, but its wall evidently nearly as thin as paper. A tail of omentum partly enveloped it, and this was much inflamed and freshly adherent. Everywhere else the peritoneum was healthy, and no indication of the formation of any bounding wall of adhesions existed. Coils of small intestine surrounded this full-to-bursting sac. The omentum was gently separated and the inflamed portion ligated and cut away. The mesentery of the appendix was carefully tied in sections, and the base of the appendix dislodged from an inverted pouch of cecum, ligated at its base, and cut away. It proved to contain at least half an ounce of very foul brown pus, but no concretion. Its communication with the cecum was closed by stricture, so that the unbroken, purulent acutely inflamed cyst was removed entire [sic]. The stump was disinfected with a 1-to-1000 bichloride solution. Two silver-wire sutures passing through the whole thickness of the abdominal walls closed the upper part of the wound, and one similar suture the lower part. The central portion was loosely packed with iodoform gauze down to the ligated stump. Dressing of iodoform and bichloride gauze over all.

At 6.40 pm, less than six hours after the operation, patient's temperature was 99.8° and pulse 80. A small quantity of morphine was given for wound pain. The dressings were changed on the third day, and a perfectly aseptic condition of wound found. This patient made a rapid and absolutely unbroken recovery, and is today perfectly well.

This is, I believe the first recorded case where an acutely inflamed unruptured appendix has been removed full of pus. Who can doubt what the result would have been in this particular case had the cyst ruptured, and the operation been delayed a few hours? Would not the opportunity for recovery have been lost had the advice so often and so recently given been followed—to delay operation until symptoms of spreading peritonitis appeared?'

References

Cope Z. *A History of the Acute Abdomen*. London: Oxford University Press, 1965.
Ellis H. The 100th birthday of appendicitis. *British Medical Journal* 1986; **293:** 1617–18.
Kelly EC. Charles McBurney. *Medical Classics* 1938; **2:** 493–538
McBurney C. Experience with early operative interference in cases of disease of the vermiform appendix. *New York Medical Journal* 1889; **50:** 676–684.

[28]

J. B. Murphy

Successful repair of a gun-shot wound of the femoral artery (1897)

Today, the routine treatment of a gun-shot wound of a major artery is repair rather than ligation. Yet ligation was the commonly performed operation in World War II and vascular repair only became relatively common in the Korean conflict. This was somewhat surprising since the first repair of a gun-shot wound of the femoral artery was successfully performed in Chicago by J. B. Murphy nearly a hundred years ago—in 1897.

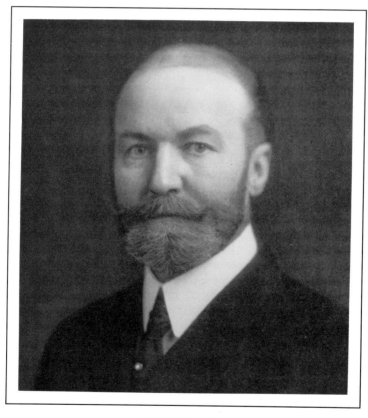

J. B. Murphy
(From L. Davis *Surgeon Extraordinary. The life of J. B. Murphy*
London, Harrap 1938)

J. B. Murphy was undoubtedly one of the most colourful characters in American surgery. Even his name reflects something of this character; he was born of humble Irish immigrants on a farm in Wisconsin and was christened plain John Murphy. However, when he went to school, he noticed the majority of the other boys had at least two initials and so, determined not to be inferior, he added the 'B'. He studied medicine at Rush Medical College, Chicago and graduated in 1879. He interned at Cook County Hospital, spent two years in Vienna under Billroth and, after being on the staff at Rush and Cook County, he became chief of surgery at the Mercy Hospital, Chicago, a position which he held until his death.

Murphy advanced surgical knowledge of almost every region of the body. He devoted much attention to the surgery of the lung and was the first in America to carry out artificial pneumothorax. He was interested in the surgery of the bone and joint, advanced our management of peritonitis and his 'button' an ingenious device for effecting intestinal anastomosis, has recently been re-introduced, now in an absorbable form.

Murphy had several minor attacks of coronary thrombosis, and at the age of 59 years, he succumbed to a major infarct.

One of his most noticeable contributions to surgery was his study of vascular anastomosis. This was based soundly on extensive and detailed animal studies. His case report in 1897 comes at the end of a long 15 page paper which details experiments which he performed in dogs, calves and sheep and in which he describes his studies on lateral repair, end to end suture and apposition by invagination of the carotid and aorta. Silk was the suture most often used and the operations were performed, of course, without the advantage of anticoagulation.

J B Murphy "Resection of arteries and veins injured in continuity—end to end suture—experimental and clinical research"

Medical Record 1897; **51**: 74–88

'Italian, peddler, aged twenty-nine. He was shot at eleven o'clock September 19th, and was brought to hospital two hours later.

Clinical history: the patient was shot twice, one bullet passing into the abdominal wall just above the great curvature of the stomach without penetrating the abdomen; the other entered Scarpa's triangle below Poupart's ligament. There was no bruit at this point or increased pulsation noticed at the time the patient was admitted to the hospital. I saw the patient first October 4th; examination revealed a loud bruit; it could be heard with the ear placed six inches from the thigh. There was no tumour and but slight increase in pulsation. The pulsation in the popliteal, dorsalis pedis, and posterior tibial arteries was scarcely perceptible. I examined the case again on October 6th and demonstrated it to a class of students. A thrill could be felt and a bruit could be heard. The latter was the loudest to which I had ever listened. The pulsation though very feeble could now be felt in the dorsalis pedis, but not in the posterior tibial.

Diagnosis: Penetrating wound of the common femoral artery about one and one-half inches below Poupart's ligament. It was decided to cut down and expose the artery, and if a penetrating wound of more than one-half of the circumference was found to make a resection and unite it end to end.

Operation: October 7 1896. An incision five inches long was made from Poupart's ligament along the course of the femoral artery. The artery was readily exposed about one inch below Poupart's ligament; it was separated from its sheath and a provisional ligature thrown around it but not tied. A careful dissection was made down along the wall of the vessel to the pulsating clot. The artery was exposed one inch below that point and a ligature thrown around it but not tied; a careful dissection was made upward to the point of the clot. The artery was then closed above and below with gentle compression clamps and was elevated, at which time there was profuse hemorrhage from an opening in the vein. A cavity, about the size of a filbert, was found posterior to the artery communicating with its calibre, the aneurysmal pocket. A small aneurysmal sac about the same size was found on the anterior surface of the artery over the point of perforation. The haemorrhage from the vein was very profuse and was controlled by digital

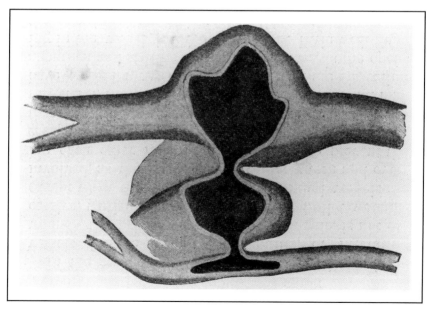

The arterio-venous aneurysm of the femoral vessels

compression. It was found that one-eighth of an inch of the arterial wall on the outer side of the opening remained, and on the inner side of the perforation only a band of one-sixteenth of an inch of the adventitia was intact. The bullet had passed through the centre of the artery, carried away all its wall except the strands described above, and passed downward and backward, making a large hole in the vein in its posterior and external side just above the junction of the vena profunda. Great difficulty was experienced in

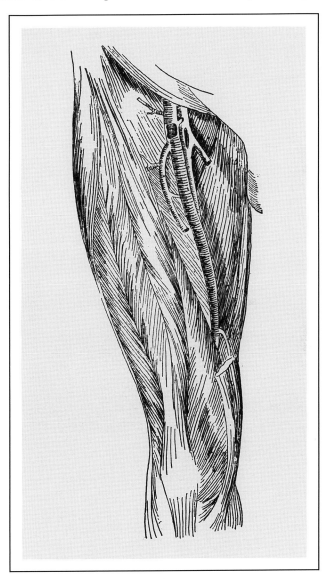

The sites of arterial and venous injury

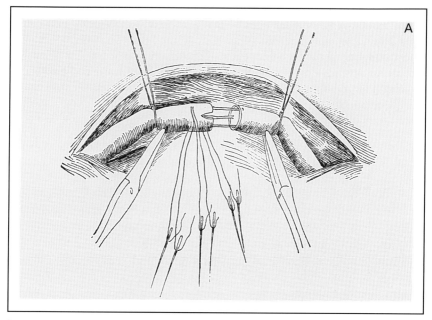

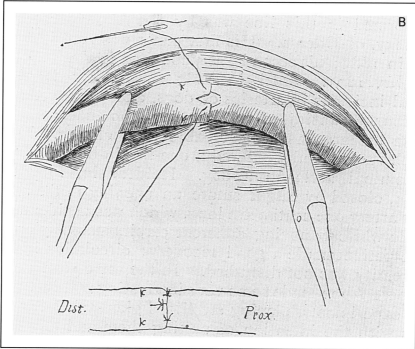

(A) and (B) steps in the arterial repair
(The operative illustrations are taken from JB Murphy *Medical Record* 1897)

controlling the hemorrhage from the vein. After dissecting the vein above and below the point of laceration and placing a temporary ligature on the vena profunda, the hemorrhage was controlled so that the vein could be sutured. At the point of suture the vein was greatly diminished in size, but when the clamps were removed it dilated about one-third the normal diameter, or one-third the diameter of the vein above and below. There was no bleeding from the vein when the clamps were removed.

Our attention was then turned to the artery. Two inches of it had been exposed and freed from all surroundings. The opening in the artery was three-eighths of an inch in length; one-half inch was resected and the proximal end was invaginated into the distal for one-third of an inch with four double-needled threads which penetrated all the walls of the artery. The adventitia was peeled off the invaginated portion for a distance of one-third inch; a row of sutures was placed around the edge of the overlapping distal end, the sutures penetrating only the media of the proximal portion; the adventitia was then drawn over the line of union and sutured. The clamps were removed. Not a drop of blood escaped at the line of suture. Pulsation was immediately restored in the artery below the line of approximation, and it could be felt feebly in the posterior tibial and dorsalis pedis. The sheath and connective tissue around the artery were then approximated at the position of suture with catgut, so as to support the wall of the artery. The whole cavity was washed out with a five per cent solution of carbolic acid and the edges of the wound were accurately approximated with silkworm-gut sutures. No drainage.

The time for the operation was approximately two and one-half hours, most of the time being consumed in suturing the vein. The artery was easily secured and sutured, and the hemorrhage from it readily controlled. The patient was placed in bed, with the leg elevated and wrapped in cotton.

A pulsation could be felt in the dorsalis pedis on October 11th, four days after the operation. There was no oedema of the leg and no pain. The circulation was good continuously from the time of the operation. The wound suppurated; drainage was inserted, but at no time did the patient's temperature exceed 100.8°F. December 8, 1896, the circulation is perfect, the wound has healed with the exception of a small superficial ulcer, one-third of an inch in diameter. The patient had not had an unpleasant symptom since the operation. January 4th, patient is walking about the ward of the hospital, has no oedema and no disturbance of the circulation.'

References

Davis.L. Surgeon Extraordinary: The Life of J. B. Murphy. London: George G Harrap, 1938.

Ellis H. Notable names in Medicine and Surgery 4th Edition. London: HK Lewis, 1983.

Murphy JB. Resection of arteries and veins injured in continuity—end to end suture—experimental and clinical research. Medical Record 1897; 51: 74–88.

Part IV
The Surgeon at Work

[29]

Lorenz Heister

Amputation of a cancerous breast (1720)

Today, we take the blessings of modern anaesthesia for granted. It is difficult for us to imagine the agonies that patients underwent in the centuries preceding the modern era, inaugurated in October 1846 at the Massachusetts General Hospital (Chapter 2).

This description by Lorenz Heister of a mastectomy which he performed in 1720, gives us a vivid idea of what major surgery comprised in those days. He discusses the careful pre-operative preparation, the mastectomy itself, performed at maximum speed, and the tedious post-operative dressings of the invariably suppurating wound (if the patient was lucky enough to survive).

Heister's case report is interesting also because it shows that times have not changed all that much in patients' attitudes to cancer. So often they try to rationalize for a cause; his patient ascribed hers to cold air on the breast when she was in a sweat 16 years before the lump appeared and while she was pregnant. All too often patients put their faith in alternative

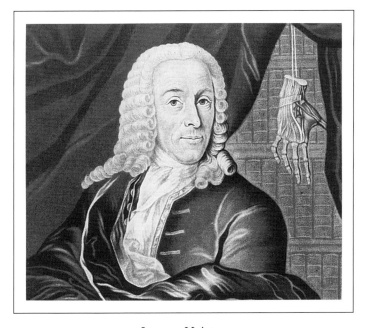

Lorenz Heister
(Reproduced by permission of the President and Council of the Royal
College of Surgeons of England)

medicine—his patient visited many quacks, who applied plasters, ointments and fomentations.

Although Heister was convinced that his patient had cancer, the description of the tumour—its mobility, the colour of the overlying skin, the bossilations, the absence of axillary metastases and the long survival of the patient suggested to Mayer and Beck that the lesion was, in fact, an example of cystosarcoma phylloides, a lesion that was not to be described till 1830 by Johannes Mueller.

Heister was born in Frankfurt am Main and proved to be a gifted student. He studied first at the University of Gieesen then Leyden and then Amsterdam, where he sat at the feet of two outstanding surgeons and anatomists, Ruysch and Rau. In 1707 he went as surgeon to the Dutch in their war against the French, returned to Leyden for further study under Bidloo, Albinus and the great Boerhaave and took his degree of Doctor in the summer of 1708. That year and the next, he returned to his duties as army surgeon.

In1710, Heister was appointed Professor of Anatomy and Surgery in the University of Altdorf in the Republic of Nurnberg, but before taking up his post he made a tour of surgical centres in Great Britain. It was during his time at Altdorf that Heister published the first edition of his great *General System of Surgery*. Shortly after its publication, Heister was appointed to the Chair of Anatomy and Surgery of the University of Helmstadt, in the Duchy of Brunswick. Later the Professorship of Botany was added to his duties and he was responsible for the establishment of its famous botanical garden. Heister remained at Helmstadt for the next 38 years. Entirely due to his influence, its school of Surgery achieved a position of great importance. Its eminence, however, disappeared rapidly after Heister's death in 1758.

Heister's great contribution to teaching was his *A General System of Surgery*, richly illustrated with 38 copper plates. It was originally written in German, in which it was published in seven editions and was also translated into ten English and three Latin editions, as well as being translated into Spanish, French, Italian and Dutch. In addition, Heister wrote a text book of anatomy which appeared in 25 editions in a variety of translations, books on eye surgery, botany and other subjects, and the magnificent collected case reports from which the present case is quoted. This report has been somewhat shortened and most of the long Latin prescriptions have been deleted.

Lorenz Heister "Medical, Chirurgical and Anatomical Cases and Observations"

London: J. Reeves, 1775

'A farmer's wife came to me, the 21st or 22nd of January, 1720, from a neighbouring village, about a mile from Altdorff, with a very cancerous right breast; she was about forty-eight years of age, of a thin habit of body, and of a melancholic temperament, had been delivered of eight children; her breast was of a prodigious size, nearly as big again as her head, very hard, unequal, and deformed, and attended with severe pains; the breast is represented, plate viii. It was of a dark brown, red colour, like a mortified part, and here and there several large bloated veins appeared; the breast was not quite round,

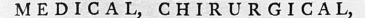

MEDICAL, CHIRURGICAL,

AND

ANATOMICAL CASES

AND

OBSERVATIONS.

By *LAURENCE HEISTER*, M. D.

Senior Profeſſor of Phyſic and Surgery in the Univerſity of HELMSTADT, firſt Phyſician and Aulic Counſellor to his ſerene Highneſs the Duke of BRUNS-WICK, Member of the Imperial Academy of Sciences, and Fellow of the Royal Societies of LONDON and BERLIN.

With COPPER-PLATES, illuſtrating the Deſcriptions in the reſpective Caſes.

Tranſlated from the German Original

By *GEORGE WIRGMAN*.

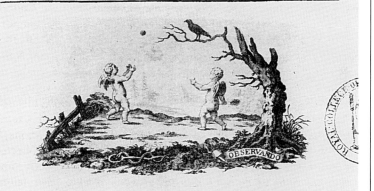

OBSERVANDO

LONDON: Printed by *J. REEVES*,

For C. HITCH and L. HAWES, and J. BALDWIN in *Pater-noſter-Row*, J. WHISTON and B. WHITE in *Fleet-ſtreet*, J. and J. RIVINGTON in St. *Paul's Church-yard*, and A. LINDE in *Catherine-ſtreet* in the *Strand*.

M DCC LV.

Frontispiece of Heister's *Medical, Chirurgical and Anatomical Cases* English edition, 1755 the left-side A, was as big as a large person's head, and next to it on the right-side B, such another substance adhered, of the bigness of a child's head, which extended itself to her right-arm as described in the figure.

Upon the inferior part of this large tumour, there were about twenty large excrescencies of a blackish colour, and of the size and form of the nipple, which I was not able to distinguish from them: these, added to the shocking aspect of the breast itself in general, rendered the appearance more horrid and frightful.

The woman was extremely weak and faint of herself, but the great weight of her breast, which weighed twelve pounds, was so troublesome when she walked, sat down, or lay in bed, pressing upon the thorax, that the respiration was so much affected, that it was with great difficulty she breathed at all; this rendered her yet more weak and faint. She complained too of a violent shooting pain in her breast, shoulders, and back, which, by contracting the thorax, contributed to produce the great anxiety and oppression she

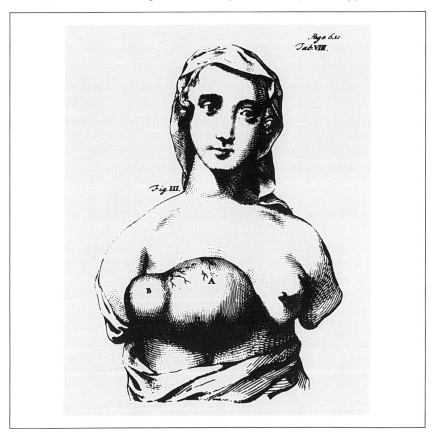

The 48 year old farmer's wife with 'a very cancerous right breast'
(From Heister *Medical Chirurgical and Anatomical Cases* 1755)

complained of in breathing: I considered and examined every circumstance, reflected upon the uncommon magnitude of the breast, and finding the tumour moveable, without any adhesion to the ribs or sternum, for I could move it with ease from side to side, upwards and downwards, nor were the axillary glands enlarged or swelled, and as she complained of no other particular disorder, I could do no otherwise than inform her friends, that it was impossible for medicine to be of any use, and that there was no other method of cure but by amputation; and that this operation would of course be attended with danger, but that if she would submit to it, there were some hopes of a cure, and of preserving her life, for without taking off her breast, she would, in all probability, soon expire with the pain, continual restlessness, oppression, and weakness.

When she heard there were hopes of saving her life, she begged of me most earnestly to do whatever I thought necessary, and I accordingly promised to take off the breast very soon; but being desirous to know in what manner she became affected with this disorder, and how, from time to time, it had increased to the present enormous size, I enquired of her, and she related to me, that about sixteen years before, during the time of her lying-in, being alone at home one day, and in a sweat, a person knocked at the door, rising, in this sweat, to see what he wanted, she perceived the cold air to strike upon her breast, and soon after observed an hard moveable lump, of the size of a hazel-nut, in the same breast, but without pain while in this state, so that she paid no regard to it, she had three children afterwards, who she suckled without perceiving the tumour to increase; but aftewards it increased gradually, and at the end of twelve years it was become as large as a hen's egg.

She now began to be apprehensive of the consequence, and had applied to many quacks, who had used, plaisters, ointments, fomentations, &c. to resolve or discuss the tumour or to bring it to a suppuration, but without success: it became bigger and bigger, till at length, her breast was as large as her head, and began to be very painful, and the more it became enlarged, the more pain it gave her: still she applied to other people of this sort for relief, used what they advised for a time, but without any benefit, but, on the contrary, the breast grew worse.

About the end of November last, another quack came to her, and promised certainly to cure her, swearing that he could soften the tumour, and bring it to suppuration, and to that intent he applied emolient cataplasms for a month, which, instead of being serviceable, had increased the pain, and the smaller tumour B, on the right side of A appeared. She was now, by this treatment, rendered so weak that she was scarcely able to walk across the room; her breast before was quite round and equal, consisting of the single tumour only. In this miserable condition she was when she applied to me.

She also informed me, that since her first lying in, she had always been troubled with various tumours in her legs, which went off gradually with her menses, and both entirely left her about a year ago, when her breast became so large.

With regard to the cure of this terrible disorder, I conceived that there was indeed no great hopes, as the tumour was of such an enormous size, which in amputation, would require so large a wound, and as the woman herself was so greatly debilitated by the constant pains and length of time she had been afflicted, that she was not able to walk.

Celsus, that excellent Roman physician, has intimated to his successors, that, in dangerous cases, it is better to try a doubtful remedy, where the least hopes of success remains, than none . . .

I thought it adviseable to proceed to the operation; not caring to defer it any longer, as the woman would become weaker and weaker, through the violence of the pain; much less could I think of putting off so considerable an operation till spring, as is customary in France, as the patient might die before the spring came, or so weak as not to be able to undergo the operation: for which reason, notwithstanding the days were short, and the weather the coldest in the year, I thought it would be dangerous to defer the operation till the spring; and accordingly, as necessity has no law, I fixed upon January 29th, for the day. I prepared every thing in the morning for the operation, the necessary instruments, namely a knife, see tab xxii. fig. 7, of my surgery; which, though pretty large, I chose for the purpose, as the breast was extremely large, and as with a large knife I could take it off more expeditiously.

I afterwards ordered such remedies to be got ready as were necessary to stop the bleeding . . .

A linen-compress to be dipped in the spiritus terebinthinae, and applied to the divided arteries; pledgets of lint strewed with the astringent powder; bovist; of diachylum plaister, spread upon linen, twelve slips a foot and an inch broad, and another piece a foot square; quadrangular soft linen-cloths folded, two rollers six yards long, and four fingers broad. I had also, in readiness, the cauterizing irons to apply to the arteries if they should bleed too violently. I ordered also the assistant-surgeon to have ready heated a quart of beer, adding three ounces of butter to it, to dip the largest bolsters in, to apply over all the other dressings, as Helvetius, in a treatise on haemorrhages, recommends this application in amputations of the breast, as of great use in preventing inflammations . . .

The whole apparatus being in readiness, I now proceeded to the operation; placing the patient in an arm-chair in the middle of the room, and standing on the right-side, somewhat backwards, that I might make the incision at the inferior part with greater convenience, which is different from the common method: I then desired an assistant to extend her right-arm and raise it up, at the same time pulling it backwards; another assistant kept her head fixed: a third stood before, who I directed to hold the diseased breast with both hands, to raise, and, at the same time, to pull it towards him, that I might with greater ease, divide it from the subjacent muscles: a fourth assistant stood on my side with the instruments and dressings, and the fifth held the cordial medicines.

I now encouraged her to behave with resolution, and taking hold of her breast with my left-hand, applied the knife to the inferior part with my right-hand, cut through the integuments, and directed the assistant who held the breast, to pull the breast towards him; I carried on the incision by the direction of the finger of my left-hand, till the breast was extirpated,which was performed in a minute.

The arteries, after the amputation, bleeding briskly, I applied to them compresses dipped in oil of turpentine, directing the assistants to make a compression upon them with their fingers: then I applied to the rest of the wound, the pledgets of lint strewed with the astringent powder, and over this a large piece of bovista, till the whole wound was covered thickly with it; over these, bolsters of tow, strewed with the astringent powder, which I redirected to be gently compressed by the hands of the assistants, till the bleeding stopped: while these dressings were applying, I gave the patient some of the cordial julep, and held the spirit for smelling to, under her nose; by which means she was kept from fainting.

The dressings I fixed with the twelve long slips of plaster, and over these I laid the large square compress, and over this two more large compresses, wetted with the hot beer and butter, and fixed the whole with a two headed roller, in the manner described, plate xxxviii. fig. I, of my surgery.

After the dressing she repeated the cordial, and was put to bed. I ordered an assistant to sit by her bed-side, to compress the dressings with his hand extended, to prevent fresh bleeding, and desired the assistants to relieve each other every two hours.

I weighed the breast afterwards, and found it to weigh twelve pounds. A few hours afterwards the blood forcing its way through the dressings, I ordered another compress to be applied, and fixed with a roller in the manner of the first, which stopped the bleeding quite . . .

February the 2nd, she was dressed again, and being tired of the julep, and having a desire for some wine, I permitted her to drink half a wine glassful of red Franconian wine at meals. I afterwards suffered her to take a glassful as she had no fever, and which agreed extremely well with her . . .

But as the discharge of matter increased, and forced its way through the dressings, I began to dress the part every day; and as there was no inflammation, omitted the compresses with the hot beer and butter, and only applied dry bolsters; about fourteen days afterwards the wound was clean, and of a red aspect, except a little place at the axilla, where there was a roundish substance, like a piece of bacon, which would not come away with the ointment, I therefore laid a piece of trochisc. de minio upon it, and dressed the other part of the wound with the following tincture:

Eff fuccin ounces i
  -myrrhae,
  -aloes, aa ounces ss. m.

After this dressing, fresh granulations of flesh sprouting forth, that foul substance was destroyed by the trochisc de minio. The fourth and fifth week the wound was dressed with the tincture, warm, only once a day, when it

[179]

began to have an healing aspect about the circumference, and skin began to be produced; and there being but a small discharge at the end of the fifth week, I dressed her but every other day; for I think wounds heal better, when the discharge is small, if dressed only every other day, than every day. At the commencement of the seventh week, the fore part was not larger than a crown-piece. To promote the cure I ordered the following powder to be strewed on the wound, applying dry lint upon it, with some emplastrum saturinum over the whole, which is a good desiccative . . .

The latter end of March some Fungous flesh appearing in the wound, which was now very small, I touched it at every dressing with some vitriolum caeruleum; and as it did not yield to this application, I applied a little of the powder of the trochisc de minio, and continued this till it was quite destroyed, which was about the middle of April; after which I dressed only with dry lint, and the emplastrum saturninum, till the 2nd of May, when I left Altdorff, at which time the wound was contracted into a very small compass.

The regimen I directed this woman to observe, was, for the first fortnight thin soup and jellies; afterwards, when she had a better appetite, I permitted veal, boiled prunes, apples and pears, and eggs boiled soft; for ordinary drink, besides the vulnerary infusion prescribed above, I suffered her to drink small beer, when thirsty; at meals, as above mentioned, I allowed her a glass of wine, and in another fortnight, permitted her to drink some Altdorff strong beer. I advised her to keep herself quiet. She was regular as to stools and urine during the whole time; and, by the end of March, had recovered her strength so well as to be able to get up and walk about, was brisk and cheerful, had a good appetite, and complained of no pain all the month of April. When I went to Helmstadt, I left directions with the surgeon to dress it with the dry lint and empl. saturninum only, till it should be healed; and a little time afterwards I was informed that she was perfectly cured, and enjoyed a good state of health. She lived several years afterwards. This cancerous breast was the largest ever extirpated or described by authors.'

References

Heister L. *Medical, Chirurgical and Anatomical Cases and Observations translated from the German by George Wirgman*. London: J. Reeves, 1775.
Meyer KK, Beck WC. Mastectomy performed by Lawrence Heister in the Eighteenth century. *Surgery, Gynecology and Obstetrics* 1984; **159**: 391–4.
Zimmerman LM, Veith L. *Great Ideas in the History of Surgery chapter 32, Lorenz Heister*. New York: Dover publications, 2nd edition, 1967.

[30]

John Hunter

1—Excision of a massive parotid tumour (1785)
2—Bony tumour of the thigh with metastases to the lung (1786)

John Hunter is rightfully regarded as the father of modern scientific surgery in the British Isles. His memory is perpetuated by the annual Hunterian lectures and the Hunterian Oration at the Royal College of Surgeons of England, where too is preserved his finest monument, the Hunterian Museum.

Hunter was the first surgeon to apply the inductive system of observation and experimentation to the study of disease. He also realized that to

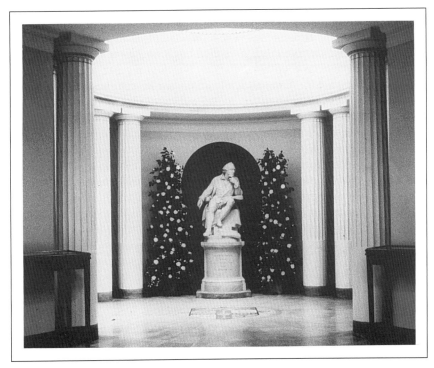

John Hunter—Statue by Henry Weekes which stands in the Inner Hall of
the Royal College of Surgeons of England
(Reproduced by permission of the President and Council of the Royal College of
Surgeons of England)

understand the effects of the disease process on the body, it is first necessary to study the form and function of the normal healthy individual. Indeed, he realized that pathological processes were 'the perversion of the natural actions of the animal economy'. His philosophy can be summed up by a famous remark he made in a letter to his friend and pupil Edward Jenner, (of vaccination fame), a copy of which is carefully preserved in the Hunterian museum, 'why do you ask me a question, by the way of solving it. I think your solution is just; but why think, why not try the experiment?'

John Hunter was born on a farm near East Kilbride, seven miles from Glasgow; his father was a grain merchant and farmer. The date of his birth was the night of the 13/14 February 1728. He observed the 14th as his birth—a date to this day celebrated annually by the Royal College of Surgeons. He was the last of ten children; his brother, William, ten years his senior, considerably influenced his early career.

John proved to be a boy who disliked his school lessons but who was keen on Natural History, which he studied in the fields and woods, a story reminiscent of Charles Darwin and Astley Cooper.

At the age of 20, John joined his brother William, who had established himself as a popular anatomy teacher in London as well as a highly successful obstetrician at the Middlesex Hospital; he was later to deliver Queen Charlotte of the future King George IV. John proved to have a flare for anatomy and became an energetic and skilled dissector. For the following twelve years he worked as assistant to William, while at the same time he studied surgery under William Cheselden and Percival Pott.

In 1760 John Hunter joined the army as Staff Surgeon and the following year, during the Seven Year War he saw active service, first in Belle Isle, off the coast of France, and then in Portugal, gaining a considerable experience in war wounds. Returning to London in 1763, Hunter set up a successful surgical practice in Golden Square and in 1768 was appointed to the surgical staff of St George's Hospital.

Hunter's first episode of what was undoubtedly angina pectoris occurred in 1773. He died on October 16th 1793 at the age of 65, while at a board meeting at St George's Hospital. At post-mortem, performed by Everard Home, his brother-in-law and surgeon on the St George's staff, demonstrated severe calcification of the arteries of the heart and brain. Hunter was buried in the crypt of the church of St Martin-in-the-Fields but the coffin was reinterred at Westminster Abbey in 1859.

Among Hunter's experimental contributions may be listed his studies on testicular descent, during which he described and named the gubernaculum testis, the demonstration of fat absorption by the lacteals, the demonstration of the blood supply of the placenta, the demonstration that the seminal vesicles do not act as a sperm reservoir and his interesting studies on grafting. These demonstrate an autograft, in which he had transplanted the spur of a cock into its comb, and allograft, in which he had grafted the testis of a cock into the abdominal cavity of a hen, and finally a xenograft, a human tooth transplanted into a cock's comb. These specimens can be seen to this day in the Hunterian Museum.

Many would regard Hunter's greatest contribution to be his museum. This he first catalogued on his return from army service in Portugal. In the next 30 years his collection grew to 13,682 specimens.

Before Hunter, museums of Natural History were collections of curiosities. Hunter's Museum was devised as a dynamic exercise in teaching. The specimens were arranged in three main categories. The first demonstrated the inter-relationship between structure and function, whether plant, animal or human. For example, the section on the nervous system demonstrated the evolutionary series from the primitive nerve chain of the earth worm to the highly developed central nervous system of man. The second group demonstrated the preservation of the race and comprised the reproductive organs and the development of the fetus. While the third series demonstrated pathological conditions.

After Hunter's death, the collection eventually passed into the custody of the Royal College of Surgeons and the specimens were moved into its buildings in 1806. On the night of 10 May 1941 the College was extensively damaged by both incendiary and high explosive bombs and over half the specimens

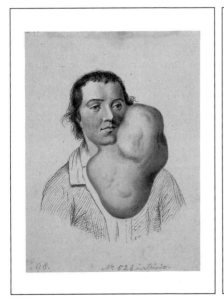 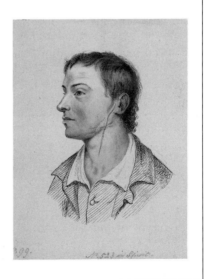

John Burley's parotid tumour   Post-operative drawing of John Burley

(From E. Allen, J. L. Turk and R. Murley *The Case Books of John Hunter, FRS* London: Royal Society of Medicine 1993, reproduced with permission of the authors and publisher)

were destroyed. However, much of the collection remains to be inspected and has been supplemented by many magnificent specimens.

John Hunter left extensive manuscript notes on his collection and these were transcribed by William Clift. He had been appointed amanuensis to Hunter in 1792, on his 17th birthday, and subsequently became the first conservator of the museum. He retired at the age of 67 in 1842.

Two of the case reports from the catalogue have been selected. Both have their specimens still on view in the Museum. The first describes a massive benign parotid tumour which was excised by Hunter without damage to the facial nerve. The second case report describes an amputation for a malignant

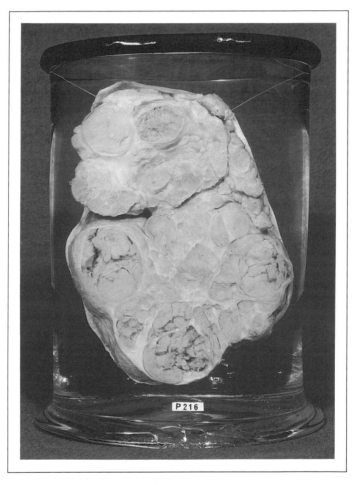

The specimen of the parotid tumour in the Hunterian Museum
(From E. Allen, J. L. Turk and R. Murley *The Case Books of John Hunter, FRS* London: Royal Society of Medicine 1993, reproduced with permission of the authors and publisher)

tumour of the femur, the patient subsequently dying with multiple pulmonary deposits. Interestingly, it appears to be the first case report in history to record pulmonary metastases.

"The Case Books of John Hunter FRS"

Edited by Elizabeth Allen, J. L. Turk and Sir Reginald Murley. London: Royal Society of Medicine, 1993

'Cases and Observations—Number 48. Tumour extracted from the neck, weighing 144 ounces

John Burley, a Rigger, thirty-seven years of age, of a middle size, dark complexion, and healthy constitution; about sixteen years ago, fell down, & bruised his cheek on the left side, above the parotid gland. It was attended with a good deal of pain, which in four or five weeks went off, and the part began to swell gradually, and continued for four or five years, attended but with little pain.

At this time it was increased to the size of a common head, attended with no other inconvenience than its size and weight. He again fell, and received a wound on its side, which gave considerable pain at first, but it got well in eight or nine weeks (This part is marked in the Drawing.) After this, the tumour increased without pain, on the lower part; as also at the basis, extending itself under the Chin to the amazing size it now appears. Lately, he had perceived that its increase is much greater than what it was some time ago: he says he can perceive it bigger every month.

The tumour is in parts the colour of the Skin, in other parts of a shining purple, where the Skin of the cheek is elongated. The beard grows upon it, and is shaved in common. When by accident it is wounded, it heals kindly, because it is only the Skin that is wounded; and has sensation in common with the Skin. It is hard to feel in some places, and in others softer, as if containing a fluid. It seems quite loose, and unconnected with the skull or lower jaw; and may be moved easily without giving pain.

The Operation was performed on Monday October the 24th, 1785. It lasted twenty five minutes, and the man did not cry out during the whole of the operation.

The tumour weighed 144 ounces.

His symptoms after the Operation were mild and gentle. Does this gentleness arise from the want of Sensibility? for the Man who had the Tumour taken out of the Calf of the leg, had his symptoms run high, and then soon sunk; and he seemed to feel the Operation as if tortured.

Cases and Dissections—Number 78. Case of a tumour in the thigh-bone which became bone: as also in the chest

A Man came into St George's Hospital November 1786, with a hard swelling of the lower part of the Thigh, as it were beginning from the knee. It appeared to be a thickening of the bone, involving in it the surrounding parts; the whole appearing to make nearly one mass.

It was then increasing very rapidly, and at this time so large as to interfere with the motion of the joint, so as to render the leg useless. The tumour was hard as bone, and seemed to be nearly equal all round the Thigh.

The man had been in perfect health in this part, 'til about five months before; and then began to feel shooting or darting pains in that part of the Thigh, which continued for four weeks; during which time he could perceive no alteration in the parts, either to appearance or to the feel: but in the fifth week, or beginning of the second month, the part began evidently to enlarge, although at first very slowly, but in the third month it increased more rapidly, and was attended with more pain as it enlarged; so that in the fifth month it was increased very considerably; and the pain was now exhausting him

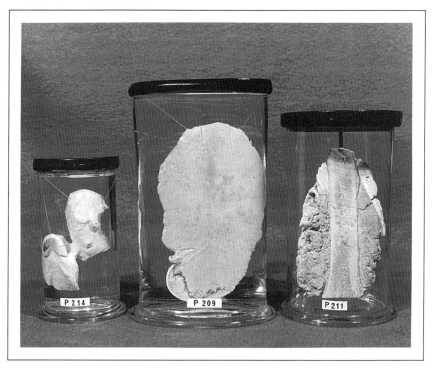

Specimens in the Hunterian Museum showing a vertical section of the lower part of the femur with a large osteoid growth around and within it (P 209); a macerated and dried section of the tumour (P 211); portions of the arch of the aorta and left auricle. On their outer surfaces are similar masses of osteoid substances (P 214)

(From E. Allen, J. L. Turk and R. Murley *The Case Books of John Hunter, FRS* London: Royal Society of Medicine 1993, reproduced with permission of the authors and publisher)

much, increasing nearly in proportion to the size; and it was thought adviseable to remove the whole, which was done. On examining the diseased part, it was found to consist of a soft substance surrounding the lower part of the Thigh-bone, of the Tumour kind, which seemed to originate from the Bone itself; into which were shooting ossifications; and as the tumour formed externally, the ossific matter formed in it; as it were keeping pace with it, the tumour becoming a nidus for bone similar to a cartilage.

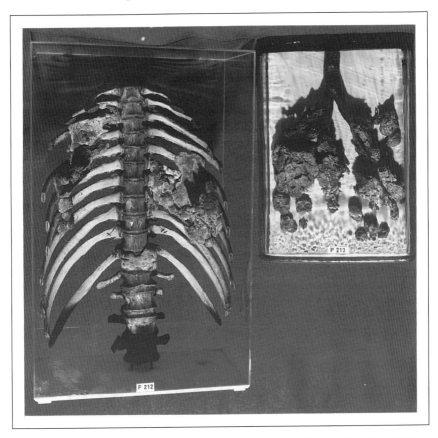

The ribs with the dorsal and some of the lumbar vertebrae—broad and thick irregularly nodulated plates of bone are attached to several of the ribs . . . a similar plate of bone is fixed on the front of the eleventh dorsal vertebra. All the bone has the same apparent structure as that of the external parts of the tumour on the femur (P 212). The dried trachea and lungs. . . . At the roots of both lungs and apparently formed in their substance are large nodulated and rough masses of spongy, but hard and heavy, bone (From E. Allen, J. L. Turk and R. Murley *The Case Books of John Hunter, FRS* London: Royal Society of Medicine 1993, reproduced with permission of the authors and publisher)

Besides this external increase of bone, there was the same internally; for the Canal as well as the whole cellular texture of the Bone was filled entirely up, so that the old bone was become compact and hard in its substance.

He went on well after the Amputation for four weeks, when he began to complain of a difficulty in breathing, but not attended with the least pain. This increased for a fortnight very much, and he then had a rigor every other day, which was supposed to be an attack of ague.

From this time he began to lose his flesh and sink gradually; his breathing being more and more difficult, and in three weeks after the difficulty of breathing came on, and seven days after the rigors, he died: living only seven weeks after the Operation.

Dissection

On examining the body, it was found that the same disposition to form Bone, which had taken place in the Thigh-bone had also affected the Thorax and its contents.

The cartilages of the Trachea were opaque, and in some places ossified: bony tumours were found in the cellular membrane of the lungs; upon the Pericardium; and some very large ones on the pleura, adhering to the ribs and upon the anterior surface of the vertebrae of the back.

These tumours, or diseased appearances, were in all the different states between soft parts and bone, so that they had not been originally formed into bone; but had been formed first of soft substance, which had afterwards been removed for osseous matter.

Besides the singularity of the disease, and appearances themselves, the seeming quick progress of the disease in the Chest is not less common or unaccountable; for when the leg was amputated, he had not the least symptom of any disease in the Chest; nor for four weeks after: and in three weeks after the first symptoms he died; in which time (from the Symptoms) we are to conclude these tumours grew. However, from reasoning, we may suppose that the appearances which were found after death, had taken place a considerable time before the Symptoms took place: yet we must allow that they could not have advanced far, and therefore their growth must have been very rapid; as indeed the increase of the Symptoms would plainly show; and if we compare this with the increase of the Thigh-bone, which was visible, we can also judge of the increase: for from the first appearance of increase, to his coming into the Hospital, was only between three and four months; and it increased more the last month than all the others.

One can figure to themselves a reason why the tumour which formed on the outer surface of the Thigh-bone might become bony, because it might acquire that disposition from the bone it surrounded: but from these Tumours formed in the Chest becoming bone, shows it was the nature of the Tumours themselves.'

References

Allen E, Turk J, Murley R. *The Case Books of John Hunter FRS*. London: Royal Society of Medicine, 1993.
Dobson J. *John Hunter*. Edinburgh: Livingstone, 1969.
Qvist G. *John Hunter 1728–1793*. London: Heinemann, 1981.

[31]

Joseph Constantine Carpue
Replacement of the nose (1816)

Surprisingly enough, replacement of the nose was carried out successfully as long ago as the 16th century by Gaspar Taliacozzo (commonly called Taliacotius) in Bologna. He published in 1597 a detailed and illustrated account of his method of raising a skin flap from the arm to replace the nose, ears or lips. The arm was kept in place by elaborate splinting until adherence had taken place and the flap was then divided from the arm. The method was little used and surgeons relied on replacing the lost nose with an artificial organ made of wood or silver.

Towards the end of the eighteenth century, reports from India described the technique of fashioning a forehead flap to replace the nose lost in fights or

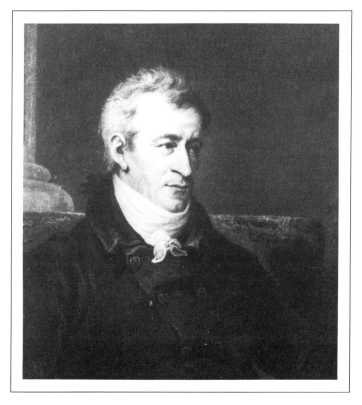

Joseph Constantine Carpue
(Mezzotint portrait engraved by Charles Turner)

by punishment which was carried out successfully by native practitioners. This came to the notice of Joseph Carpue who, in 1814 and 1815, performed two successful operations to restore a lost nose. The first patient was an army officer who had lost his nose either from syphilis or from the mercury used in its treatment. A forehead flap was fashioned and stitched around the nasal defect. The viability of the flap gave some initial anxiety, but this recovered and the cosmetic result was good. The second

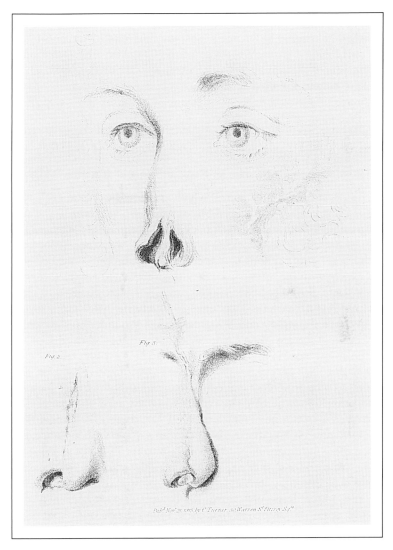

Captain Latham—showing the deformity of the nose and its repair
(From J. C. Carpue *An account of two successful operations for restoring a lost nose* London: Longman, 1816)

patient (described below) was another army officer whose nose had been lost in battle.

Carpue published his results in 1816 in a monograph entitled *An account of two successful operations for restoring a lost nose from the integuments of the forehead in the cases of two officers of His Majesty's army: to which are prefixed historical and physiological remarks on the nasal operation; including descriptions of the Indian and Italian methods.*

Carpue was born in 1764 in Hammersmith. He was a Catholic and at first considered entering the church. He did not begin his surgical studies until 1796, when he entered St George's Hospital and studied under Sir Everard Home. In 1798 he became a member of the Company of Surgeons and the following year was appointed to the surgical staff of the Duke of York's Hospital, Chelsea. He died in 1846.

J C Carpue "An account of two successful operations for restoring a lost nose from the integuments of the forehead"

London: Longman, Hurst, Rees, Orme and Browne, 1816

'At the battle of Albuera, in Spain, which was fought on the 16th of May, 1810, the right brigade of General Stuart's division was sent to the support of the Spaniards, who were driven back from the heights they occupied on the right of the line; and, while charging the enemy with the bayonet, a body of Polish horse lancers coming up unperceived (on account of the heavy storm of rain, which, with the smoke from the firing, prevented anything from being distinctly seen), their flank was turned, and they were charged in the rear. Some of the regiments, in consequence, were almost wholly destroyed, the enemy giving no quarter, and slaughtering the wounded and fallen.

At this time, Captain (then Lieutenant) Latham, of the third foot, seeing one of the colours of his regiment in danger of being taken from the ensign who carried it, by four of five of the lancers, sprung to the spot; and, in attempting to seize the colour, he lost an arm by a sabre-cut. Still persevering, with the other hand, he tore the colour from the staff; but not before he received five wounds, one of which took off part of his cheek and nose. One of the lancers now charged him through the others, and with his lance, hit him with such force in the groin, as to throw him to the distance of some yards, almost in a state of insensibility, but still with the colour in his possession.

A body of British dragoons at length approaching, the lancers made their escape; and, immediately afterward, the fusileer brigade coming also upon the ground, some of the men of that corps found the colour under the body of Captain Latham, whom they supposed to be dead. The finders sent the colour to his regiment, saying, they had found it under one of its officers, who was killed.

Through some mistake, Ensign Walsh, who carried the colour, was at first mentioned as the officer who saved it, and whom it was found under: but

Mr Walsh, who, after being severely wounded, had been made prisoner, was, the next day, on the retreat of the French, left behind, and at liberty to rejoin his regiment; and it was then discovered by whom the colour had really been preserved. On this occasion, the brother officers of Captain Latham, in acknowledgement of his gallantry, presented him with a medal, which, through the sanction of His Royal Highness the Commander-in-Chief, he is permitted to wear. His Royal Highness was, at the same time, pleased to promote him to the rank of Captain.

The transaction above related, having recommended Captain Latham to the notice of the Prince Regent, His Royal Highness, as will afterward be more particularly mentioned, was pleased, in the month of January last, to place that gentleman under my care.

In the state in which the nose was left by the sabre of the enemy, all the interior was exposed. Exclusively of the disagreeable appearance produced, Captain Latham suffered from repeated colds and inflammations.

The right side of the alae remaining, the patient preferred a cicatrix in the middle of the nose to an amputation of the sound part. I consulted my friends, Mr Astley Cooper, Mr Sawrey and Mr Anderson, surgeon to the captain's regiment, who were of opinion with myself, that the integuments taken from the forehead would unite with those which covered the side of the nose.

I made an incision on the forehead, as in the former case; as also similar dissections. On making the dissection of the forehead, there was a very considerable haemorrhage; so much so, that I was compelled to tie an artery. When the flap hung down, instead of the part appearing purple, as in Case I, an artery bled as freely as the temporal artery when opened. This, however, subsided; and there was no occasion for a ligature.

The parts were brought into contact, as in Case I, by means of five ligatures: the only difference was, that the right side of the integuments, instead of being received into an excavation, was brought into exact contact; and that the lip was not divided, but the lower part of the septum dissected away, and the new part brought into contact, and detained there by ligature.

Adhesive plaster was applied to the forehead, as before, and the usual dressings.

The patient had some fever in the first night, but with a little sleep. More haemorrhage than in Case I.

Second day. Free from pain. Little fever.

Third day. The part felt very uncomfortably. Removed the dressings. Much inflammation. Inner part of the integuments united; but the skin did not adhere. Cut away the ligatures, and brought the skin together by adhesive plaster.

Fourth day. Considerable suppuration from the internal parts. Forehead in a very good state. Adhesion complete between the eyebrows. . . .

Tenth day. The skin, which had been disunited by the swelling of the parts, restored to perfect union. (Oedema not so considerable; and, in this case, pressure seems of advantage.)

In six weeks, forehead completely healed.

At the end of two months, oedema less considerable; and afterward continued to decrease. There remains, however, an oedematous disposition.

On the 7th of October, in the presence of Messrs. Warren and McLochlin, I performed the second part of the operation, which consisted in making a longitudinal incision under the top of the nose, and then, continuing the dissection across the bridge, under the new nose. After this, I dissected away a considerable portion of the under surface of the new nose, and then made a longitudinal incision in the new nose, so that the new nose was made to fit as nearly as possible the excavation I had made in the old nose. I now brought the longitudinal incisions of the old and new noses exactly in contact, passed two silver pins through the integuments, and united them by the twisted suture. Then I applied adhesive plaster to the remaining parts. Forty-eight hours after the operation, I removed the dressings; and, finding that a perfect adhesion had taken place, I withdrew the pins, and applied adhesive plaster. A little suppuration followed from the lower pin, but of no consequence. The parts were perfectly recovered in two days. In ten days, the time usually allowed, complete adhesion had taken place. A dissection of the new nostril remains to be made.

Captain Latham he enjoined me not to conclude this account of his Case, without recording some particulars of the generosity and benevolence of His Royal Highness, the Prince Regent, which are intimately connected with it, which it is his pride to acknowledge, and for which he feels that he can never be sufficiently grateful. It will appear, from the following copy of a letter which I had the honour to receive from Major-General Bloomfield by the hand of Captain Latham, that his Royal Highness not only condescended to place that gentleman under my professional care; but, further, to direct me to provide, at his Royal Highness's private charge, for the personal accommodation of my patient, during the cure. In addition to this liberality, since the operation has been performed, and it has been proper that Captain Latham should have the benefit of the air, His Royal Highness has been pleased to cause one of his carriages to attend him daily for that purpose.

(Copy)

Major-General Bloomfield is commanded by the Prince Regent that Mr Carpue will give the unfortunate case of Captain Latham, who will hand him this letter, his utmost attention and care. The particular gallantry displayed by Captain Latham has invited an additional interest in His Royal Highness. Major-General Bloomfield is further commanded to request, that Mr Carpue will make such arrangements for the accommodation of Captain Latham as may give facility for the professional attendance of Mr Carpue, the whole expenses of which will be defrayed by His Royal Highness.'

(The Prince Regent ascended the throne as George IV on the death of his father, George III in 1820. HE.)

Reference

Carpue JC. *An account of two successful operations for restoring a lost nose from the integuments of the forehead*. London: Longman, Hurst, Rees, Orme and Browne, 1816.

Baron Guillaume Dupuytren

Baron Guillaume Dupuytren and his contracture (1834)

It is remarkable that a condition as common as Dupuytren's contracture, which affects some 15 per cent of the male population over the age of sixty, and which is such an obvious 'spot' diagnosis, was only well documented in 1833. It was Dupuytren who demonstrated, by post mortem dissection, that the disease was a lesion of the palmar fascia. His description reads 'this fascia was tense, retracted and shortened, from its lower portion were given off kinds of cords which passed to the diseased finger'. The overlying skin and the underlying tendons, joints and bones were all sound. He noted that 'the greater number of individuals affected by this disease have been obliged

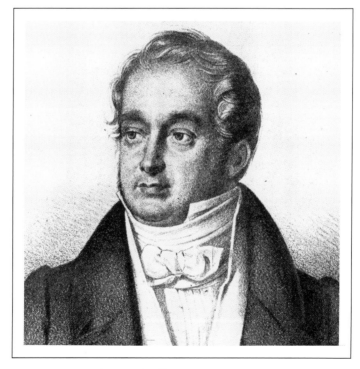

Baron Guillaume Dupuytren
(Reproduced by permission of the President and Council of the Royal
College of Surgeons of England)

to make efforts with the palm of the hand, or frequently to handle hard bodies'. He noted the condition in coachmen, masons and ploughmen.

Guillaume Dupuytren (1777–1835) rose from poverty to be the leading surgeon of France, a baron of the Empire and a millionaire. He commenced his medical studies in Paris at the age of 18 in the early days of the French Revolution. For weeks at a time he lived on bread and cheese and it is said that he was forced to use the fat of the subjects in the dissecting room to make oil for his lamp! By 1808 he was appointed surgeon second class to the Hôtel Dieu and by 1815, (the year of the battle of Waterloo), he was appointed Surgeon-in-chief.

Dupuytren was a man of superabundant energy. His daily ward rounds were at six in the morning and seven in the evening. His daily clinical lectures were given to three or four hundred pupils. He was an excellent teacher, an operator of the utmost self-control and a shrewd clinical observer. He was a pioneer of excision of the lower jaw and of the cervix of the uterus, of lumbar colostomy and of ligation of the subclavian artery. He was also dogmatic, averse to criticism, convinced of his own superiority, ambitious and a tyrant to his residents. He showed little consideration for the suffering poor under his care. He was called by his contemporaries 'the first of surgeons and the least of men'.

At his death following a stroke at the age of 57, he left an enormous fortune amassed by his own efforts as the acknowledged leading French surgeon of his day.

Dupuytren's lecture at the Hôtel Dieu in 1833 was published in the *Lancet* in London the following year in accordance with its editor, Thomas Wakeley's, plan to give publicity to the teachings of famous centres from around the world. Here follows the case report from this paper:-

Guillaume Dupuytren "Clinical lectures on surgery delivered by Baron Dupuytren during the session of 1833. Permanent retraction of the fingers produced by an affection of the palmar fascia"

Lancet 1834; 2: 222

'Cases of Contraction of the Ring and Little Fingers completely Cured by Division of the Palmar Aponeurosis

Case 1—In 1811, M L., wine-merchant, having received from the South a great deal of wine, was desirous to assist his workmen in arranging the casks in the store. While endeavouring to raise one of the casks, which was very heavy, by placing his hand under the edge of the stave, he felt a sensation of cracking and a slight pain in the palm of his hand. For some time the part remained stiff and sensible, these symptoms soon went off, and he paid little attention to the state of his hand. The accident was nearly forgotten, when he perceived that the ring-finger commenced to contract towards the palm of his hand, and could not be extended as much as the other fingers. As there was no pain, he neglected this slight deformity. By degrees the disease advanced, and made a sensible progress each year, so that in 1831 the little and ring fingers were completely flexed and applied to the palm of the hand; the second phalanx was folded on the first and the extremity of the third applied to the middle of the ulnar edge of the palmar surface. The small finger was firmly flexed on the palm of the hand; and the skin of this part was folded, and dragged towards the retracted fingers.

The patient, annoyed by seeing this deformity getting daily worse, consulted several surgeons, who all said that the disease existed in the flexor tendons, and advised their section as the only remedy; but some would cut both tendons, whilst others proposed to divide only one.

The moment I saw the man's hand I recognized the affection of the palmar fascia, declared the disease was not situated in the tendons, and that a few incisions practised in the aponeurosis would be sufficient to restore entire freedom of motion to the finger.

Operation: The hand of the patient being firmly fixed, I commenced the operation by making a transverse incision nearly an inch long, opposite the

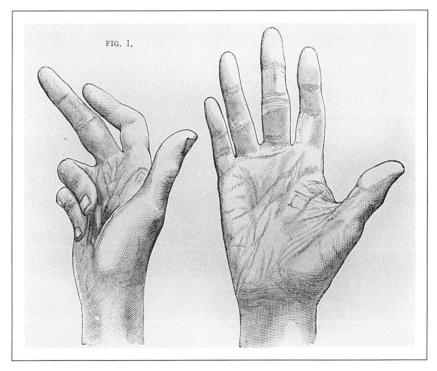

Dupuytren's contracture
(A woodcut from William Adams *On contraction of the fingers (Dupuytren's and Congenital contractions) and Hammer-toe* London: Churchill 1892)

metacarpophalangeal articulation of the ring finger; the bistoury divided first the skin and then the palmar fascia, with a cracking sound perceptible to the ear; after this incision the ring-finger recovered its position and could be extended nearly as completely as ever.

As I was desirous to spare the patient the pain of a new incision, I attempted to prolong the division of the fascia by gliding the bistoury deeply under the skin towards the ulnar edge of the hand, in order to free, if possible, the little finger, but this attempt failed.

I was in consequence obliged to make another transverse incision opposite the articulation of the first and second phalanx of the little finger, which enabled me to detach it from the palm of the hand, but the rest of the finger remained obstinately fixed towards this part. A new incision, however, divided the skin and fascia opposite the metacarpal joint of the finger, to give it some slight liberty; finally, a third transverse cut was made opposite the middle of the first phalanx, and immediately extension of the finger was easily accomplished; this proved clearly that the last incision had divided the point of insertion of the fascial process. The wounds were simply dressed with dry lint, and the fingers kept in a state of extension by a suitable apparatus.

Progress of the case—Next day, little pain; merely some uneasiness from the continued extension. On the following day the back of the hand was slightly oedematous from the pressure of the apparatus, which was clumsily made; another was applied, but the state of irritation continued, great pain set in, and the hand became much swollen. Not wishing to remove the machine applied to extend the fingers, I ordered the hand to be bathed continually with Goulard's solution, which gave considerable relief. On the 15th the lint was removed, and we found some suppuration had set in; the hand was still swollen and painful. Extension was continued to the same degree as formerly, and the cold lotion applied. On the 16th the swelling had abated considerably, the fingers remained stiff, and suppuration was fully established, 17th. The symptoms were more favourable, and the extension could be increased somewhat without determining any pain. Finally, in the course of some days the swelling of the hand disappeared, and the wounds were healed on the 2nd of July.

Case 2—The subject of this operation was a coachman aged about 40. Several years back his fingers began to contract, especially the ring-finger. When he came to the Hôtel Dieu, the fingers were so much flexed that they nearly touched the palm of the hand; and this part formed numerous folds of skin, the convexity of which was turned towards the fingers. When we attempted to extend the fingers, we felt a cord stretching from them to the palm of the hand; both hands were affected by the disease, which could not be mistaken, from its history, and the symptoms before us. When the hand was seized, and the fingers moved, the tension of the fascia became manifest.

I immediately divided with a curved bistoury the skin and fascia by two incisions, one at the base of the ring-finger, in order to cut the two slips of the fascia passing to it; the second time, and at the point where its base joined the palmar aponeurosis.

After three incisions the ring-finger recovered very nearly its normal position; though little blood was lost the patient himself felt weak, I therefore deferred operating on the left hand until another day. It is unnecessary to pursue the history of this case any further, as the treatment and success were exactly similar to the case already mentioned to you.'

References

Dupuytren G. Hôtel Dieu, Paris Clinical lectures on Surgery delivered by Baron Dupuytren during the session of 1833. Permanent retraction of the fingers produced by an affection of the palmar fascia. *Lancet* 1834; 2: 222–5.

Ellis H. *Notable Names in Medicine and Surgery* 4th edition. London: Lewis, 1983.

[33]

Alfred-Armand-Louis-Marie Velpeau

Excision of a recurrent tumour of the breast (1856)

Breast cancer has been studied from the very earliest days of surgery and, before any surgeon could even dream of tackling other cancers such as stomach, bowel or lung, operative techniques which would fulfil modern criteria were being developed for its cure.

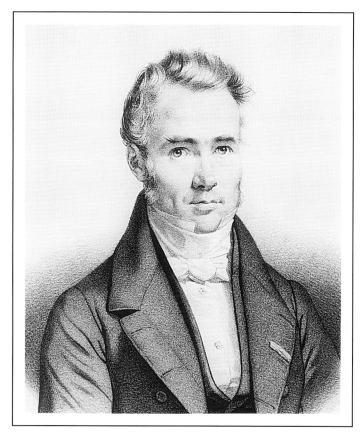

Alfred-Armand-Louis-Marie Velpeau
(Reproduced by permission of the President and Council of the Royal
College of Surgeons of England)

The growth, ulceration and spread of breast cancer, with ultimate inevitable destruction of the patient, was obvious to the earliest observers. In Hippocrates we read 'A woman in Abdera had a carcinoma of the breast and bloody fluid ran from the nipple. When the discharge stopped she died'.

Celsus, in the first century AD, recorded early attempts at surgery for this disease:- 'Some have used caustics, others the cautery, other cut them out with a knife . . . Notwithstanding they have returned and occasioned death.'

By the middle of the 17th century, total mastectomy, using the amputation knife and the cautery, was pictured graphically in the *Armamentarium Chirurgicium* of Scultetus, published in Ulm in 1653, eight years after the death of its author.

Heister's vivid description of an amputation of the breast in 1720 is quoted in Chapter 29.

Probably the first surgeon to advise *en bloc* excision for breast cancer was Jean Louis Petit (1674–1750) of Paris, who wrote 'The roots of cancer were the enlarged lymphatic glands; that the glands should be looked for and removed and that the pectoral fascia and even some fibres of the muscle itself should be dissected away rather than leave any doubtful tissue. The mammary gland too should not be cut into during the operation. Where the integuments are . . . joined to the cancer there is little hope to expect a perfect cure if they are not both clearly extirpated together'.

Over the next century, many surgeons advocated complete mastectomy together with axillary clearance. In 1784, Benjamin Bell of the Edinburgh Royal Infirmary, in his six volume textbook, wrote 'Even when only a small portion of the breast is diseased, the whole mamma should be removed. The axillary glands should be dissected by opening up the armpit but as much skin as possible should be preserved'.

In 1825, Sir Astley Cooper, in his *Lectures on the Principles and Practice of Surgery*, wrote 'It will be sometimes necessary to remove the whole breast, where much is apparently contaminated; for there is more generally diseased than is perceived and it is best not to leave any small portion of it, as tubercles reappear in them. . . . If a gland in the axilla be enlarged, it should be removed, and with it all the intervening cellular substances. . . . If several glands in the axilla be enlarged, their removal does not succeed in preventing the return of the disease'.

By 1844, Joseph Pancoast of the Jefferson Medical College in Philadelphia was advising still more radical surgery; involved muscle should be removed, even affected portions of ribs should be resected with the cutting forceps or a saw and 'such of the axillary glands as are supposed to be scirrhous, or are even indurated and enlarged, should be taken away'.

Of course, these operations were being performed without any form of anaesthesia. Once the blessing of ether had been introduced by Morton in 1845, more leisurely surgical dissection became possible.

A landmark in the history of breast disease was the publication in Paris in 1854 of *Traité des maladies du sein et de la région mammaire*, which appeared two years later in English translation as *A treatise on the diseases of the breast and mammary region* published in London and translated by Mitchell Henry, Assistant Surgeon at the Middlesex Hospital. This monumental work of nearly 600 pages, was based on a vast clinical experience and illustrated by numerous detailed case reports, of which the one to be quoted is an excellent example.

Alfred-Armand-Louis-Marie Velpeau was born in 1795, the son of a master blacksmith. He commenced his medical studies in Tours at the age of 20 and continued his studies in Paris two years later. At the age of only 25, he published his treatise on surgical anatomy, which passed through three editions and numerous translations. He dallied with obstetrics, published a book on the subject, but returned to his first love of surgery. For 34 years he was Professor of Surgery in the Faculty of Medicine of Paris and surgeon to the Charity Hospital of Paris. His reputation depended more on his great powers as a teacher, writer and clinical observer rather than being a particularly brilliant operator. His other publications included a thesis on trepanation of the skull in head injuries, a text book of operative surgery and a treatise on embryology. He died in Paris in 1868 at the age of 73.

A Velpeau "A treatise of the diseases of the breast and mammary regions"

London: Sydenham Society, 1856

'Encephaloid tumour extirpated three times, and eventually radically cured—In the year 1841, I was consulted, at the Rue St George, by Madame V-, a lady of 56 years of age, stout, strong, well-formed, but very nervous; who stated to me that a year previously one of my colleagues in the hospitals of Paris, had removed a tumour from her right breast, and that shortly after the cicatrization of the wound, a second one had made its appearance. The new tumour existed on the lower and external border of the cicatrix. It was as large as a hen's egg and had a large base; its summit, shaped as a globular projection, or like the top of a penny roll was of a reddish violet colour, and fluctuating. Venous branchings covered its surface, and lost themselves at the root in the rest of the region. This projection rested on a somewhat thickened base, tolerably firm, like lardaceous scirrhus, which was continuous with the glandular tissue below the cicatrix, and preserved considerable mobility on the surface of the chest. The axilla was free, and there was no swelling in any other situation. The tumour which had been removed in the year previously was preserved. It was formed by a central nucleus of encephaloid appearance, and by a lardaceous mass, which appeared to form a sort of shell for this substance. The whole also seemed to be enveloped in a tolerably thickish layer of sound tissue, so as to make it probable that no altered structures had been left behind. This examination, it is true, filled me with alarm; but Madame V-'s general condition, and the, as yet, circumscribed limits of the disease, left no room for hesitation. I recommended and performed a fresh operation a week later.

The tumour was removed like a slice of melon, in an ellipse of sound tissue. Abundant suppuration followed, and the cicatrization of the wound was not complete for about six weeks. The morbid structure presented all the characters of encephaloid tissue. It was softened, fungous, medullary, reddish, and vascular in the external projection; lardaceous, homogeneous, and brownish in some parts; and everywhere continuous with a thick layer of mammary tissue, which I had removed along with it.

Eighteen months after this operation, Madame V- applied to me again for a third tumour, which had made its appearance in the right breast. This new growth was situated above and to the outer side of the last cicatrix, in front of the anterior border of the axilla. Somewhat smaller in size than the last tumour, it bore, however, a striking resemblance to it in all other aspects. The cicatrices were intact; there was nothing as yet in the axilla; the general health was not more disordered than previously, and there being no sign of cancerous cachexia observable, M. Marc Moreau and I came to the conclusions that a third operation should be performed. This operation, which the patient cheerfully agreed to, and which she supported, like the others, with great courage, was simple, and easily executed. The natural stoutness of the patient, and the suppleness of the healthy parts, allowed the lips of the wound to be brought in contact. Six weeks elapsed before cicatrization was complete, but no serious incident occurred. This time the cure was complete. I have seen Madame V- every year since, and for long past she has ceased to dread the return of the disease in her breast. At the present time, 1853, she continues in good health. It need hardly be added, that the last tumour exactly resembled the others in its anatomical composition and texture, and in the appearances which it presented at the bedside.

M. Roux, indeed, states that he on one occasion succeeded after six returns of the disease.

Even when we cannot obtain a radical cure, it may still be useful in some patients to remove the cancer afresh. I have in this way prolonged the lives of several for a considerable number of years. A lady at Brest, operated upon for the first time in 1842, and subsequently a year later, by M. Foulloi, came to Paris in 1845, when I removed from her a fibro-plastic cancer, situated on the cicatrix of the old wound. The patient, having perfectly recovered from this third operation, returned to Brest, but came up again a year later with a fresh tumour, which I again extirpated and easily cured.

In 1852 she submitted to a fifth operation, and her general condition was such as not entirely to destroy all hope of a radical cure.

It is, at any rate, incontestable that this patient would have died six or eight years ago, if a fresh operation had been declined after the first return of the disease.'

References

Ellis H. The treatment of breast cancer: a study in evolution (Bradshaw Lecture 1986) *Annals of the Royal College of Surgeons of England* 1987; **69**: 212–5.
Velpeau A. *A treatise on the diseases of the breast and mammary region*. Translated from the French by Mitchell Henry. 1st English Edition. London: Sydenham Society, 1856.

[34]

John Hilton

Injuries to the musculo-cutaneous nerve (1863)

In early 1862, John Hilton, of Guy's Hospital, London, completed a series of lectures at the Royal College of Surgeons entitled 'Rest and Pain'. These he published in book form in October 1863 and it is still in print today. In it, Hilton emphasized two great surgical principles: the first is the value of long and continuous rest to damaged tissues and the second is the diagnostic value of pain, especially when a deep knowledge of anatomy can be applied to the elucidation of this symptom.

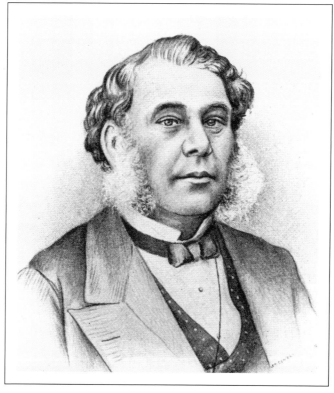

John Hilton. About the year 1867, when he was 60 years
of age
(Reproduced by permission of the President and Council of the
Royal College of Surgeons of England)

Hilton was born in 1807 in a rural village in Essex, about 50 miles to the North-East of London. He entered Guy's Hospital as a pupil at the age of 17 and from the age of qualification until he was 38 years of age, he was a lecturer in Anatomy. This laid the foundation of his deep knowledge of the human body which coloured the rest of his career. Even when appointed as assistant surgeon at Guy's, he continued to lecture on Anatomy. His long surgical career ended when he died from gastric cancer at the age of 71.

Rest and Pain still provides both education and interest to the Clinician. Hilton construed the word 'rest' in its widest sense and he wrote:- 'a man received a blow on the chest from a fall upon the part . . . I could find no fracture of the ribs; but I observed that the patient had a most worrying wife. I suggested to the physician that the sole cause of the pain, was in all probability, produced by the patient constantly moving the injured or bruised soft parts by using his chest and lungs in speaking. All I recommended was that he should hold his tongue and have his chest bandaged. I requested that his wife should not say a word to him. From that time, he got quickly well by local rest'.

How many of us have treated an injured chest by recommending that both husband and wife should hold their tongues?

To illustrate Hilton's literary style, I have chosen these two case reports from his book:-

J Hilton "Rest and pain. A course of lectures on the influence of mechanical and physiological rest in the treatment of accidents and surgical diseases, and the diagnostic value of pain"

London: Bell, 1863

'Injury to the Musculo-Cutaneous Nerve by a bullet

I had once an excellent opportunity of seeing a well-marked case of injury to this musculo-cutaneous nerve. A lieutenant in the Navy was at Lagos, fighting with the natives. He jumped ashore with his sword in his right hand and ran with his men up to a stockade. Although he was struck once or twice, he went forward; presently his sword-arm dropped; he could grasp his sword in his hand with great vigour, but could not bend or raise his forearm. This gentleman, before he returned to his boat, received seven balls, of which some went through the right side of his chest. When I saw him in London, I removed a bullet from his leg, and he then explained to me the nature of the injury which he had received in his arm. This made one of the most precise experiments that you could possibly conceive upon the external cutaneous nerve. The bullet had bruised or severed the nerve, causing a paralysis of the biceps and brachialis anticus; both muscles were wasted, whilst the other muscles of the arm were well developed; a curious-looking depression was thus produced in the arm over the wasted muscles. In order to bend his right forearm, he used to place his left hand behind his right, and forcibly jerk the forearm into the flexed position. The sensibility of the skin over the ordinary distribution of the external cutaneous nerve was destroyed. He had consulted the late Mr Guthrie as to giving up his appointment in the Service and he subsequently came to me with the same object. I said I did not think the nerve had been divided. It might have been; there was no doubt it was seriously injured. I advised him, whether the nerve were divided or not, to retain his commission, as the probability was greatly in favour of its being ultimately repaired. He obtained leave of absence for two or three years and wore his arm in a short sling. I met him three years afterwards in Piccadilly, when he flourished his stick in the air with his right arm and said he was ready for anything. I asked him how long he had been getting well and he told me 'About two years and a half'. His arm was quite strong, and the wasted muscles had nearly regained their normal size. The power of grasping and moving the fingers which this gentleman retained after his injury left no doubt that the median and ulnar nerves were uninjured. This was a well-defined injury, that marked very completely the distribution of the musculo-cutaneous nerve. This gentleman, as a captain in Her Majesty's Service, is now receiving his reward for his courage and his wounds.

Exostosis pressing upon the Musculo-Cutaneous Nerve

I may mention another fact with regard to the same nerve. Four or five years ago a boy came to me at Guy's Hospital, with his arm contracted, and suffering a good deal of pain in the course of the external cutaneous nerve. On careful examination, I found a simple exostosis pressing upon this nerve as it passed through the coraco-brachialis muscle. He had several other similar exostoses at different parts of his body, but they did not pain him. I cut down upon the exostosis to which I have specially refered and removed it. He had no longer any pain, and was soon able to move his arm freely.'

References

Hilton J. *Rest and Pain. A Course of Lectures on the Influence of Mechanical and Physiological Rest in the Treatment of Accidents and Surgical Diseases, and the Diagnostic Value of Pain.* London: G. Bell and Sons, 1863.
Keith A. *Menders of the Maimed.* Chapter 2 page 18. *John Hilton's Principles of Treatment.* London: Oxford University Press, 1919.

[35]
Jaques-Louis Reverdin
Myxoedema following thyroidectomy (1882)

Goitres occur, of course, in iodine deficient areas of the world—areas as far away from the sea as possible and particularly in elevated inland zones. In the United Kingdom, this situation occurs in Derbyshire. As a young Resident Surgical Officer in Sheffield the author became well acquainted with 'Derbyshire Neck'. In the USA it is the Mid-West, and to this we owe the expertise in thyroid surgery of the Mayo brothers in Rochester Minnesotta and of Crile in Cleveland. Medical visitors to Nepal and to the Ethiopian highlands will be struck by the high incidence of large thyroid masses, and this was certainly my experience as examiner, many years ago, in the University of Addis Ababa at the Princess Tsahai Memorial Hospital—(renamed the Black Lion Hospital of the People's Socialist Republic of Ethiopia). In Europe, the inland mountains of Switzerland were famous for their endemic goitres—now all but abolished,

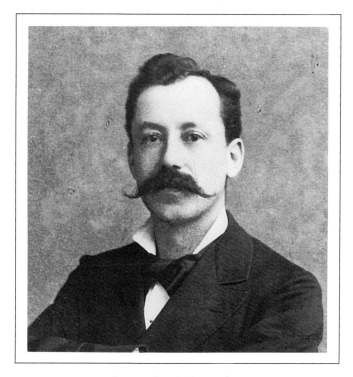

Jaques-Louis Reverdin
(Courtesy of Dr Guy Saudan, Pully, Switzerland)

as in other civilized areas, by iodination of table salt. And it was in Switzerland that so much of the surgery of the thyroid gland was developed.

On September 15th 1882, Jaques-Louis Reverdin reported to a meeting of the medical society of Geneva hitherto undescribed symptoms following goitre surgery. In the report of that meeting, published on the 15th October in *la Revue médicale de la Suisse Romande*, he wrote:-

Two or three months after the operation the patients have presented for the most part with a state of weakness, pallor, anaemia and, in two of them, oedema of the face and hands with albuminuria; in one case there was pupil contraction, melancholy and prostration, and in another the facies resembled that seen in cretins.

(Translation by H E)

At the same meeting, it was recorded that Theodor Kocher of Berne reported that he had had a case of depression and weakness following thyroidectomy.

This report of Reverdin was the first well documented occurrence of hypothyroidism following thyroidectomy.

The following year, Reverdin, together with his cousin and personal assistant, Auguste Reverdin, documented in meticulous detail the results of his first 22 goitre operations. These were spread over three issues of *la Revue médicale* and ran to no less than 122 pages of text; a great contrast to what authors might expect to be able to publish today! No less than five of their patients developed these untoward symptoms. All had undergone total thyroidectomy. Reverdin pointed out that these features resembled the syndrome described by Sir William Gull of Guy's Hospital, London in 1874 and later termed myxoedema by William Ord of St Thomas's Hospital.

Reverdin made the important recommendation that only partial removal of the thyroid gland should be performed.

Kocher, after the Geneva meeting, had gone back to study his own cases and reported a similar phenomenon at the 12th Congress of Surgeons in Berlin later in 1883 and termed this syndrome 'cachexia strumipriva', while Reverdin introduced the much more apt title of 'operative myxoedema'. Here we should record that Kocher received the Nobel Prize for medicine for his work on thyroid surgery; well deserved certainly, but perhaps it should have been shared with Reverdin.

Jaques-Louis Reverdin was born in Geneva in 1842, studied medicine in Paris and served in the Franco-Prussian War of 1870 as a surgeon during the siege of Paris. In 1879 he established a private clinic with his cousin and the two worked together for the next 20 years until his retirement in 1910. In his retirement he made a considerable reputation for himself as an entomologist. He died in 1929. His name is preserved eponymously in Reverdin's needle, still much used, especially by gynaecologists.

In this abstract from his massive paper is his description of one of his five examples of operative myxoedema.

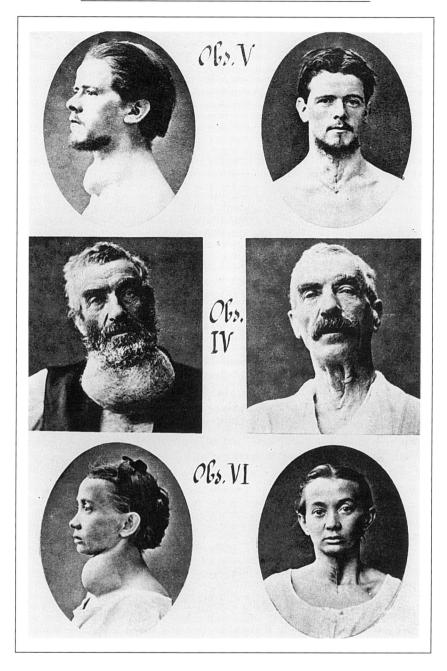

'Before and After' photographs of patients with massive goitre operated upon
by J. L. Reverdin. Note the vertical neck incision
(Courtesy of Dr Guy Saudan, Pully, Switzerland)

Jaques-Louis Reverdin and Aug. Reverdin "Note on 22 operations for goitre"

Revue Médicale de la Suisse Romande 1833; 3: 309–364

'Observation XI Miss S Juliette, 33 years old. Operated 15th November 1880 for cystic goitre; total removal. Healing complete in 10 days . . . She came to see me on the 4th December perfectly well having lost the discomfort produced by her tumour; general as well as local condition good.

At the end of the second month, she felt fatigued, she had become pale and she no longer had either strength or spirit; she was not aphonic, but she might suddenly completely lose her voice; moreover her voice had changed in tone and had become deeper . . . She came to see me on 7th February 1881. She seemed to me to have a pronounced anaemia but there were no other symptoms apart from the ones I have listed; I prescribed iron.

In spite of this her condition did not improve; on the contrary during the next three months it got worse without changing its characteristics; only the hands which became heavy, sluggish and clumsy; during the whole of the Winter she could hardly work, above all in carrying out fine tasks such as crochetting; she did not experience any tingling but the hands felt dead. Her memory became like her hands, numbed and idle; she was obliged to think for a long time before remembering what she had to do.

At the beginning of the summer she began to improve and little by little she regained her normal health but she did not feel completely herself until the end of the year . . . I reviewed Miss S on many occasions; in February 1883 she felt very well; in May she reported to me that her health was excellent, that all her troublesome symptoms which had bothered her for a year had completely disappeared; her colour restored, she could walk easily and could work as before; the only thing that persisted was the change in her voice which still troubled her when she was tired or cold, and her poor memory . . . I found on inspection that her complexion was slightly yellowish and that her eyelids appeared a little thickened; at all events she was notably fatter.'

(Translation by H E)

References

Mayer R. Jaques-Louis Reverdin. *Revue Médicale Suisse Romande* 1980; **100:** 1013–1041.

Reverdin J-L, Reverdin A. Note sur vingt-deux opérations de goitre. *Revue Médicale Suisse Romande* 1883; 3:309–364

Saudan G. Jaques-Louis Reverdin (1842–1929) and his cousin Auguste (1848–1908) of Geneva; or how surgical practice prevailed over experimental physiology. *Journal of Medical Biography* 1993; **1:** 144–150.

[36]
William Stewart Halsted
A swallowed foreign body; bladder stones; gunshot wound of the skull (1884)

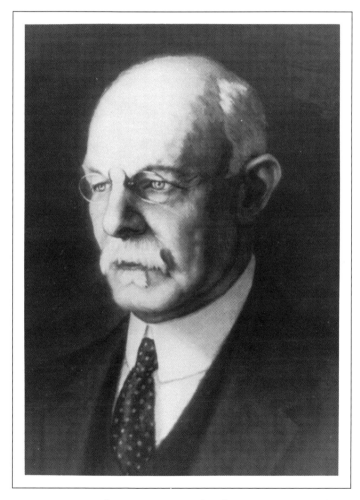

William Stewart Halsted in 1922
(From J. O. Robinson *Silvergirl's Surgery—the Biliary Tract* Austin,
Silvergirl 1985, with the author's permission)

William Stewart Halsted is recognized as one of the father figures of American surgery. He was born in 1852 in New York City to a wealthy family of English origin. Educated at a private school and at Yale, he graduated head of his class at Columbia University at the age of 25. After interning at Bellevue, he spent two years in Europe studying at Vienna, Leipzig and Würzburg. At the age of 29, he plunged into a busy New York practice as attending surgeon to the Presbyterian, Bellevue and Roosevelt hospitals.

Then, his career faced ruin. Experimenting with cocaine as a local anaesthetic agent, he became addicted to the drug and, for a while, had to discontinue practice. Although probably never quite the same, he was able to overcome his addiction, transferring to Baltimore at the age of 35 to the newly opened Pathological Laboratory at Johns Hopkins.

In 1889, at the age of 37, he was appointed Surgeon in Chief, joining a distinguished staff that included William H. Welch, Simon Flexner, and Walter Reed. Here he founded a school of surgery that produced a stream of distinguished graduates which included John M. T. Finney, Harvey Cushing and J. C. Bloodgood among others.

Halsted died following an operation for gallstones in 1922 at the age of 70.

Halsted's contributions were extensive, particularly in the fields of intestinal anastomosis, hernia repair, arterial ligation for aneurysm, and wound healing. He pioneered a technique of meticulous and painstaking haemostatic surgery. His name is now applied eponymously to the operation of radical mastectomy, which he first reported in the *Bulletin of The Johns Hopkins Hospital* in 1890.

The breadth of his general surgery can be seen by the following three brief case reports, recorded in a single contribution. These span the fields of ear, nose and throat, urology and neurosurgery!

W S Halsted "Removal of foreign bodies"

New York Medical Journal 1884; 39: 226–227

'Case 1—A piece of fibro-cartilage removed from the esophagus by external esophagotomy

At Ward's Island, July 23 1882, a Hungarian aged thirty-three swallowed at dinner a piece of food which became arrested in his esophagus a little below the cricoid cartilage. The resident physicians were unsuccessful in their attempts to dislodge it. They obtained, however, a fragment which, submitted to microscopical examination, proved to be fibro-cartilage. The patient was said to have experienced great difficulty in breathing for several hours, and then to have become quite tolerant of the foreign body, but to have been unable to swallow even liquids.

July 25th—The foreign body, indistinctly definable by palpation of the neck, was believed to be lodged in the esophagus, just above the sternum, projecting more to the right side than to the left. An incision, extending from the middle of the thyroid cartilage to the interclavicular notch of the sternum, was made parallel with the anterior border of the sterno-cleido-mastoid muscle. The oblique jugular vein was drawn toward the median line. The middle thyroid vein in the upper angle of the wound was doubly ligated and divided. The common carotid artery, crossed by the omo-hyoid muscle, rolled up into view. The foreign body was readily mapped out through the esophageal walls, and over it was stretched the recurrent laryngeal nerve. An incision an inch and a quarter long was made into the esophagus, parallel with and posterior to the nerve, and the foreign body, measuring $1.5 \times 1 \times 1$ inch, was removed with a vulsella. The wound in the esophagus was united by sulphurous-acid (*sic*) catgut, and the integument by silk sutures. An idoformized peat dressing was applied. A few days later the patient was clandestinely served with blackberries by missionaries to the island, which interfered with union by first intention, but otherwise did not hinder his prompt recovery.

Case II—Three calculi, each with a portion of a soft catheter as a nucleus, removed from the bladder by lateral lithotomy at one operation

The patient, a Finn, about thirty-five years old, had been in the habit of evacuating his paralysed bladder with a soft catheter. One day the catheter broke off in his bladder, and a piece, believed to be two or three inches long, was left behind.

He subsequently regained the power of his bladder, and applied, six or eight months after the mishap, at Ward's Island, for relief of frequent and painful micturation. A stone was detected by Thompson's searcher. In consideration of the history, it was believed to be advisable to practice the cutting operation. The patient had such a short perineum that the finger, introduced into the bladder, could ascertain the number and shape of the stones. These were carefully seized with the forceps so as not to be crushed, and removed.

The patient's convalescence was somewhat protracted because of a cystitis perpetuated by a few fragments, which he eventually passed per urethra.

Each calculus contained a piece of the catheter, its point being distinctly visible in one of them.

Case III—A portion of a bullet removed from the diploe and cranial cavity

Mr H.U.G. aged fifty-two was admitted to the Chambers Street Hospital, May 9 1883, for a self-inflicted pistol shot wound of the head.

A small circular scalp-wound was found on the right side, two inches and a half below the sagittal suture and one inch in front of the external auditory meatus. The reflexes were normal, and there was no paralysis; the intellect was perfectly clear.

A crucial incision was made through the scalp. The external table was found depressed, and at the bottom of the depression there was a hole one quarter of an inch in diameter and about one inch behind the bullet wound in the soft parts. A probe, passed obliquely backward through the hole, detected the foreign body, which was not visible.

Thereupon certain fragments of the external table were removed, and the bullet was revealed, lying between the two tables, and projecting somewhat into the cranial cavity. Upon its extraction, a slightly depressed fragment of the inner table was withdrawn.

The wound was dressed antiseptically, and closed with a continuous catgut suture. Union took place by first intention throughout, except where the incisions crossed one another—viz, at the point of entrance of the bullet—and here there was a very slight necrosis of the approximated corners of the flaps.

The bullet had split upon the outer table of the parietal bone; one fragment entered the diploe and cranial cavity; as described, and the other passed through a mirror and was found behind the bureau.'

References

Halsted W S. Removal of foreign bodies. *New York Medical Journal* 1884; 39: 226–7.
Kelly E C. William Stewart Halsted. *Medical Classics* 1938; 3: 385–509.

[37]
Sir John Bland-Sutton
Splenectomy for wandering spleen (1893)

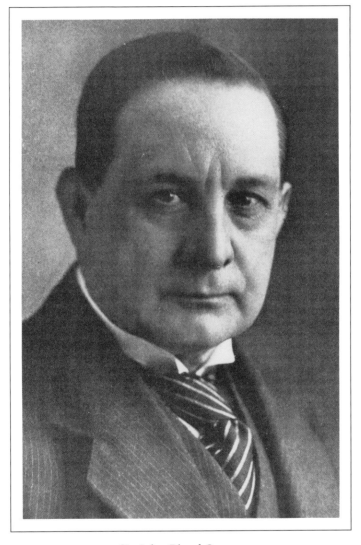

Sir John Bland-Sutton
(From W. R. Bett *Sir John Bland-Sutton* Edinburgh: Livingstone 1956,
reproduced with permission of the publisher)

Whether Andriano Zaccarello did or did not remove the greatly enlarged spleen of a lady of 24 in Naples in 1549 is a subject of debate among surgeons and medical historians. However, there is no doubt at all that the first successful splenectomy for a pathologically enlarged spleen was carried out by Jules Péan at the St Louis Hospital in Paris in 1867. This was in a girl of 20 with an enormous splenic cyst (see chapter 4).

Recurrent torsion of a 'wandering' spleen is a rare condition, yet this pathology features among a number of the early splenectomies with recovery; these were reported by Martin in Berlin in 1877, in a woman of 31, and Czerny in Heidelberg, in a woman aged 30, the following year.

The first report of splenectomy for torsion in this country was recorded by John Bland-Sutton in 1893.

Bland-Sutton was born in Enfield, Middlesex, in 1855. His was a humble background, his father was a market gardener, and Bland-Sutton never lost his cockney accent. In 1878 he enrolled as a student at the Middlesex Hospital, qualified four years later with the conjoint diploma and the LSA, and proceeded to the FRCS in 1884. He distinguished himself in the Anatomy Department at the Middlesex and also carried out many dissections of rare animals obtained from the London Zoo. In 1886, he was appointed assistant surgeon and lecturer in anatomy at the Middlesex and, in 1896, became surgeon to the Chelsea Hospital for women. Always a general surgeon, with a particular expertise in abdominal surgery, he also became one of the founders of gynaecological surgery in the United Kingdom; he was especially adept in the surgery of uterine fibroids.

He had an enormous private practice. He always used silk for ligatures and sutures, which he purchased in balls one mile in length. When asked how much money he earned, he replied that he was not sure. However, he reckoned that each ball of silk represented £10,000 in fees and he remarked that he used quite a number of balls of silk each year!

Bland-Sutton became President of the Royal College of Surgeons in 1923 and was made a Baronet in 1925. He died in 1936 and, at his wish, his ashes were placed in an urn in the gallery of the museum of the Bland-Sutton Institute of Pathology at the Middlesex Hospital.

J Bland-Sutton "A case of axial rotation of a wandering spleen: Splenectomy: Recovery"

Transactions of the Clinical Society of London 1893; 26: 46–49

'In March 1892, Mr W Rees placed under my care Alice F., aet. 22 years, on account of an abdominal tumour. The patient was a tall thin woman, and mother of one child. She had suffered during the preceding two years from occasional attacks of pain in the left side. Three months before admission the patient noticed a 'lump' in the left side of the belly. This 'lump' appeared shortly after a miscarriage. Fourteen days before this woman was sent to me she was suddenly seized with acute abdominal pain, vomiting, diarrhoea, and difficulty in micturition. Coincident with this attack, the swelling in the belly became larger.

When admitted into the Middlesex Hospital a large tumour was found in the left half of the belly, lying between the costal arch and iliac fossa. It appeared to extend backward into the loin, but it was so movable that it could be depressed into the pelvis or carried over to the right loin.

Thinking the tumour might be a movable kidney, hydronephrotic from kinking of the ureter, observations were made upon the urine. The quantity and quality of the urine did not support this view, and Mr Henry Morris, who kindly saw the case with me, demonstrated that it could not be the kidney, because this organ could be felt quite easily on account of the laxity of the belly-wall. Another suggestion, that it might be an ovarian cyst with a long pedicle, was not entertained after an examination of the pelvic organs. Among the various forms of abdominal tumours I felt that the diagnosis really rested between a wandering spleen and a hydatid cyst of the omentum. As the patient was suffering much pain it was decided to examine the abdomen through an incision. The exploration was carried out on March 21 by an incision in the middle line between the umbilicus and the symphysis of the pubes. The tumour was found to be a very large spleen, and on examining the pedicle it was found to be twisted. I endeavoured to untwist it without withdrawing the spleen from the belly. This was not satisfactory, so I enlarged the incision, drew out the spleen (very tenderly, for it was so engorged as if only too willing to burst), straightened the pedicle, and returned it. The spleen at once slipped upwards to its place in the left hypochondrium. The wound was closed in the usual manner. Next morning, in response to my inquiry, 'How do you do?' the patient replied 'I have lost that dreadful pain which I have had for more than a fortnight'.

The wound united by first intention; the swelling gradually diminished and retreated under the costal arch, and on April 4 the patient was discharged at her own request, wearing a carefully adjusted belt.

It should be mentioned that the spleen at the time of the operation seemed to have made one and a half revolutions, and it is of interest to observe that the symptoms produced by this movement were identical with those indicating acute axial rotation of an ovarian tumour. Six weeks after the operation the patient reported herself. On examining the abdomen I could not find any tumour, and the splenic dullness was of about the usual extent.

On July 7 the patient came again to the hospital in great distress. Nine days previously the lump again appeared quite suddenly, but caused her no inconvenience until July 4, when she was seized with intense pain in the belly and back, vomiting, diarrhoea, metrorrhagia and inability to lie down in bed. On examining her it was clear that the spleen had again descended. The patient was readmitted. Mr Henry Morris kindly saw the patient, and was of opinion that the spleen should be removed. This opinion was endorsed by Drs Cayley and Kingston-Fowler and Mr J. W. Hulke. The patient willingly assented. In order to show the wandering propensities of this spleen it will be sufficient to state that on July 9 it was in the right iliac fossa, obscuring the caecum and in contact with Poupart's ligament. On July 10 it was in the left iliac fossa in contact with Poupart's ligament, and on July 12 it was in the pelvis in contact with the uterus. As far as could be judged it did not seem to move about entirely by its own weight. For example, when the woman turned to the left side the spleen would sometimes fall to the left side, but quite as often it would move to the right, as though carried up by the intestines, like a boat on the crest of a billow.

On July 12 splenectomy was performed. I reopened the abdomen through the scar of my former incision, and found the spleen lying in the pelvis, its upper extremity being partially hidden by coils of small intestine. On removing it from the belly the pedicle was found to be twisted through three complete revolutions; on this account, as well as from the large size of the veins, it resembled an exceeding thick umbilical cord. The pedicle was transfixed and tied in two halves with plaited silk. For security an encircling ligature was placed around the pedicle a centimetre below the point of transfixion; the spleen was cut away, and the wound closed in the usual manner. The patient was treated on exactly the same plan as after ovariotomy. For three days after the operation the temperature and pulse were as follows: temp 99°, pulse 104; temp 100°, pulse 96; temp 99°, pulse 92, and then became normal. She never exhibited an unfavourable symptom, and left, convalescent, August 5, twenty-five days after the operation.

A perusal of the recorded cases of splenectomy shows clearly enough that success depends in a large measure on the treatment of the pedicle. I selected moderately thin but very strong plaited silk, rendered aseptic and preserved in absolute alcohol.

The spleen weighed sixteen ounces, and differed slightly in shape from the normal organ. The anterior border presented only a shallow notch, and explained why we were unable to recognize definitely the splenic nature of the swelling before undertaking an exploratory operation. Before removing the spleen I attempted to ascertain the existence or otherwise of a spleniculus or spleniculi, but failed to find one. Nearly every foetus possesses a spleen and at least one spleniculus. Sometimes as many as five spleniculi are present, and occasionally, especially when the viscera are transposed, the spleen is represented by a number of spleniculi clustering together like a bunch of grapes, or widely separated, reminding one of asteroids. Although I failed to find a satellite spleen, its absence must not be regarded as proved. Had I recognized a spleniculus my intention was to avoid removing it with the main spleen, in the hope that perhaps it would have taken on compensatory hypertrophy, as is occasionally the case with accessory thyroids.'

References

Bett W R. *Life of Sir John Bland-Sutton, Bt.* Edinburgh: Livingstone, 1956.
Bland-Sutton J. A case of axial rotation of a wandering spleen: Splenectomy: Recovery. *Transactions of the Clinical Society, London* 1893; **26**: 46–49.

[38]

Robert Jones

Location of a bullet by X-rays (1896)

There can be few other discoveries in the Physical world that have had such an immediate and sensational effect on the practice of Medicine than the discovery of X-rays. The speed with which this invention was applied to the practical problems of diagnosis was truly phenomenal. Within weeks the first X-ray pictures of fractures and foreign bodies had been taken all over the

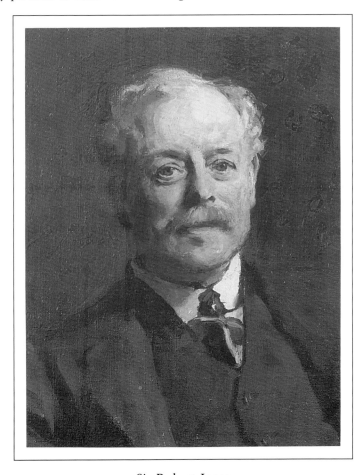

Sir Robert Jones
(Reproduced by permission of the President and Council of the Royal College of Surgeons of England)

world, and within a few months, the first journal devoted to the subject had been published.

The discovery of X-rays was made by Wilhelm Conrad Röntgen (1845–1923), then aged 50, and Professor of Physics in the small German University of Würzburg. Like many other physicists, he was experimenting with the newly discovered rays that were emitted when an electric current was passed through a vacuum tube, which had been devised by Crookes and Lenard. On the evening of the 8th November 1895 he noted that a screen coated with barium platino-cyanide, which lay on a nearby bench, became brightly fluorescent. Passing his hand between the vacuum tube and the plate, he noticed that this cast a shadow on the plate, as did other objects such as pieces of metal. Summoning his wife, he put her hand in front of the plate and photographed the resultant shadow of her hand bones and her wedding ring—the first X-ray had been taken! From the very first, Röntgen had shown the possible application of these new rays in medical diagnosis.

By the 28th December, he was able to present to the Würzburg Physical-Medical Society a written report on the important characteristics of his new rays, which could pass easily through materials such as wood and paper but not through substances such as metal and bones. Röntgen (his name is often misspelt Roentgen), entitled his paper 'Eine neue Art von Strahlen' (on a new ray) diffidently, he proposed that these mysterious emanations should be called 'X-rays'. His paper was communicated to members of the society and appeared almost at once in the Vienna newspapers. By the 6th January 1896, a full account appeared in the *London Standard*, which transmitted a world cable on the subject and pointed out its possible clinical importance. The following day, the first X-ray photograph for clinical purposes was made by Alan Campbell Swinton, an electrical engineer in London. Within a few months, *Archives of Clinical Skiagraphy* appeared, edited by Sydney Rowland, then still a medical student at St Bartholomew's Hospital, London. This journal is still being published as the *British Journal of Radiology*.

Most deservedly, Wilhelm Röntgen was awarded the Nobel Prize for Physics in 1901. We should also not overlook that the early pioneers working with these new rays, both physicists and physicians, often soon developed an annoying dermatitis of the hands and many of them went on to become victims of multiple skin cancers and of aplastic anaemia; martyrs in the development of the new science of Radiology.

The newly discovered rays (which Kolliker proposed promptly to call 'Röntgen rays'), were put to work almost at once by surgeons in the localization of foreign bodies and the diagnosis of fractures. Internists were more tardy; some even seemed to think it was an intrusion on the clinical methods of inspection, palpation, percussion and auscultation of the thorax to add an X-ray of the chest!

Publications soon appeared on the practical application of X-rays. The first I have discovered was published in the *Lancet* on February 22, 1886 by Robert Jones and Oliver Lodge of Liverpool. It is quite remarkable that in the space of a couple of months an X-ray machine was built, cases dealt with, a paper prepared and publication achieved. One wonders if such a phenomenon could occur today.

Sir Robert Jones (1857–1933) was a remarkable man and one of the father-figures of orthopaedics in the United Kingdom. He was born in the little town of Rhyl in North Wales, qualified at the age of 21 and was appointed to the staff of the Royal Southern Hospital in Liverpool at the early age of 30.

A great influence on his early life was his uncle, Hugh Owen Thomas, who had, of course, invented the Thomas splint. Thomas's father and forefathers represented generations of medically unqualified 'bone setters' who had practised their art in Wales.

Robert Jones developed a vast experience as surgeon to the canal being constructed between Liverpool and Manchester by teams of, mostly Irish, labourers. He organized a chain of hospitals to deal with the many serious injuries which were encountered. His organizational experience stood him in good stead in World War I when he established an orthopaedic service in the British army, eventually becoming a Major-General. The introduction of the Thomas splint by Robert Jones on the Western front for the treatment of compound fractures of the femur reduced the mortality of this injury from 80 to 20%. During the war he was responsible for training a great number of young American army surgeons in the United Kingdom.

Oliver Lodge, the second author of the paper, was at that time Professor of Physics at University College Liverpool. He went on to become one of the leading physicists of the early twentieth century.

Robert Jones and Oliver Lodge "The Discovery of a bullet lost in the wrist by means of the Roentgen rays"

Lancet (February 22) 1896; i: 476

'A boy aged about twelve years was brought to me by Dr Simpson of Waterloo, Liverpool, having shot himself in the left hand just above the deep palmar arch. The wound was enlarged, but the bullet could not be found, and it was thought injudicious to prolong the search in view of the important structures in the vicinity unless one possessed a clue to its position. Professor Lodge kindly consented to take a photograph and the position of the bullet was very clearly outlined. It lies against the base of the third metacarpal bone over its articulation with the os magnum. This is, I think, the first photograph taken of a bullet embedded in a wrist—in this case considerably thickened as a result of inflammation. It will now be quite easy to await subsidence of inflammatory action. The photograph was taken in the presence of Mr Houlgrave, who succeeded Dr Simpson in the treatment of the case. Arrangements are being completed for fitting up a department for the employment of Roentgen's rays at the Royal Southern Hospital.

[223]

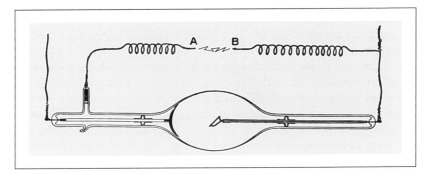

Diagram of an early X-ray tube

Note by Professor Oliver Lodge—The patient was brought to my laboratory by Mr Robert Jones, with a pellet of lead lost in his left hand or forearm. Two preliminary short exposures to Roentgen rays indicated that the metal was not in a fleshy part readily penetrable by those rays, but was probably embedded among the bones of the wrist. The difficulty consisted in the opacity

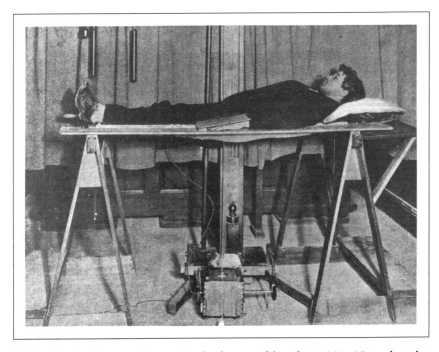

Methods of taking a radiograph of a fractured hand in 1901. Note that the X-ray machine is under, and the plate rests on top of, the hand
(F. H. Williams, *The Röentgen Rays in Medicine and Surgery* New York: Macmillan 1901)

of those bones. I therefore took a tube with large electrodes made and exhausted by my assistant, Mr E E Robinson, containing potash, so that its vacuum could be adjusted to the best value, and arranged a magnet to concentrate the inside cathode-rays on a definite part of the glass, which phosphoresces and acts as the source of the rays, the rays spreading from each point of the glass in all directions. The boy was comfortably seated at a table his palm down on an aluminium-protected Edwards' isochromatic half-plate, nine inches vertically below the vacuum tube, and rather more than two hours' exposure was given. The coil used was an ordinary Ruhmkorff, giving about two inches spark at most, and it was excited by five storage cells. The vacuum was such that a one-inch spark in air was usually preferred to the tube. The result was to bring out the wrist-bones clearly and to show the position of the pellet.'

The X-ray which accompanied this short article reproduced poorly in the original publication. Its subtitle read:-

'Roentgen radiograph of the left wrist of a lad aged 12 years showing a small bullet which had been lost in it. The bullet is located between the base of the middle metacarpal bone and the os magnum. Taken by Professor Oliver Lodge FRS after two hours exposure to a well exhausted home-made vacuum tube excited by a small ordinary coil. The sensitive plate was an Edward's isochromatic, nine inches distant from the vacuum tube, screened from light by sheet aluminium.'

References

Jones R, Lodge O. The discovery of a bullet lost in the wrist by means of the Roentgen rays. *Lancet* 1896: i: 476.
Watson F. *Life of Sir Robert Jones*. London: Hodder and Stoughton, 1934.

[39]

Sir Peter Freyer

The Freyer prostatectomy (1902)

Until the end of the 19th Century, the patient with urinary retention due to prostatic hypertrophy faced a life of misery—daily catheterization, either by the doctor or by the patient himself or, if this failed, a leaking, smelly, suprapubic tube; death resulted from chronic urinary tract infection and renal failure. Practically everything that could be tried, was tried. Hemlock, Ergot, Strychnine, Mercury, Iodine and Bromide were prescribed; prostatic massage, galvanic current, intra-prostatic injection of iodine or silver nitrate, dilatation of the prostatic urethra, castration and vasectomy were all tried and abandoned.

Perineal prostatectomy had its origin in the inadvertent or deliberate avulsion of fragments of the prostate during perineal lithotomy. As a definitive

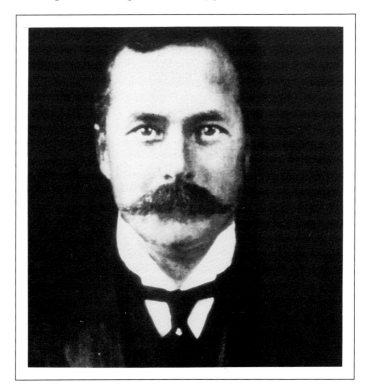

Sir Peter Freyer
(Portrait at the Institute of Urology and Nephrology London. Courtesy of the Dean, Dr F. D. Thompson)

operation, it was pioneered in the 1890s in the USA by George Goodfellow and popularized by Hugh Young of the Johns Hopkins Hospital, Baltimore.

Suprapubic removal of portions of the prostate was performed by Theodor Billroth in 1885 and this approach was developed particularly by William Bellfield of Chicago (1886), Arthur Ferguson McGill of Leeds (1887) and Eugene Fuller of New York (1895). Despite the work of these surgeons, suprapubic prostatectomy remained a neglected subject until Peter Freyer, in a series of papers and monographs, popularized the operation so that today, suprapubic enucleation of the prostate with bladder drainage through a large suprapubic tube (probably one of the reasons for Freyer's undoubtedly good results) is eponymously entitled 'The Freyer Prostatectomy'.

Peter Freyer (1852–1921) qualified from Queen's University, Belfast in 1874 and was awarded the gold medal of the year. He joined the Indian Medical Service as a surgeon, rose to the rank of Colonel and became particularly skilled in the use of the lithotrite in the crushing of bladder stones. A successful operation with this instrument upon Bahadur Ali Khan, the Rajah of Rampur, was rewarded with a lakh of Rupees and a magnificent present of jewellery, much to the dismay of his military superiors. He returned to London in 1896 and was soon appointed to the staff of St Peter's Hospital in London, then, as today, the only specialized urological hospital in the United Kingdom. He was a skilful and speedy surgeon and his excellent results attracted a large private practice. In 1920 he reported 1,625 prostatectomies with a mortality of only 5%. He was knighted in 1917.

Freyer claimed, quite wrongly, that he and only he had introduced total removal of the prostate and indeed, claimed that the essential feature of his operation was that he removed the whole prostate and its capsule from its adventitial sheath. Both these claims were patently not true and the journals of the time are filled with the acrimonious claims and counter-claims of Freyer, Fuller of New York, Mayo Robson of Leeds and others. However, the publicity given to the operation by the controversy, as well as Freyer's numerous lectures, articles and books, made the operation of suprapubic prostatectomy widely known and did Freyer himself little harm. Indeed, during the controversy, Peter Freyer quoted Sidney Smith who wrote 'that man is not the discoverer of any art who first says the thing; but he who says it so long and so loud and so clearly that he compels mankind to hear him'.

A typical example of Sir Peter Freyer's forceful style of writing is given by the following case report:-

Peter Freyer "Clinical lectures on stricture of the urethra and enlargement of the prostate"

2nd edition, London: Baillière, Tindall and Cox 1902, Page 111

'This gentleman, aged seventy-five, on the advice of the late Dr Cos, of Reading and Dr Philip, of Boulogne, came from France to consult me on

September 2, 1901. About fourteen years ago, having for several months previously suffered from severe prostatic symptoms, he was advised to pass a catheter to empty his bladder nightly on going to bed. A severe attack of cystitis ensued and since then he had never passed urine except through a

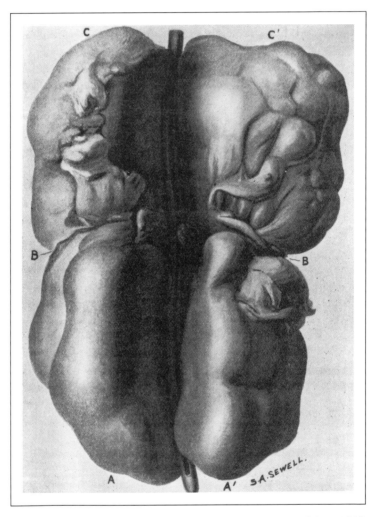

Showing upper aspect of enormous prostate, weighing 10½ ounces, removed from patient aged seventy-five; exact size. The catheter indicates position occupied by the urethra. Portion A, A^1, B, B^1, lay in bladder; that, B, B^1, C, C^1, outside bladder, between pubic arch and rectum. C, C^1, anterior aspect lying against triangular ligament

(From P. J. Freyer, *Clinical lectures on stricture of the urethra and enlargement of the prostate* 2nd Edition. London: Baillière, Tindall and Cox 1902)

catheter. For the last few years he has had frequent attacks of haematuria, often very profuse, intense pain at times, great scalding in passing the catheter, which he has had to employ latterly every half-hour day and night . . .

I introduced a long coudée catheter, No. 9 English scale, with some difficulty, 14½ inches entering before the urine flowed, and drew off 3 ounces of foetid urine, containing much pus and some blood. The prostate was felt enormously enlarged *per rectum*, but fairly soft. The kidneys were probably affected. The patient was in great agony.

On September 6, assisted by Mr H Frankling, I performed total extirpation of the prostate. I commenced by passing a coudée catheter, and drew off 2 or 3 ounces of urine of a fearful stench. The bladder was washed out repeatedly with solution of permanganate of potash. It was then distended

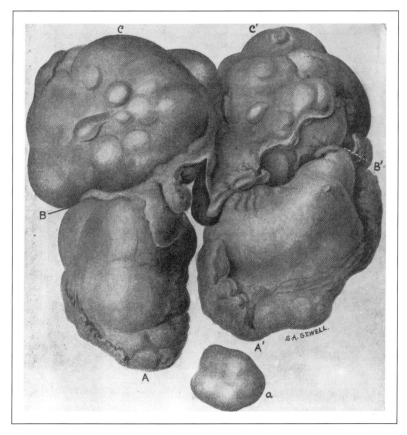

Showing under aspect of the same prostate. A, B, A¹, B¹, growth from lateral lobes projecting into bladder. C, B, C¹, B¹, prominences felt per rectum; a, adenoma detached from prostate
(From P. J. Freyer, *Clinical lectures on stricture of the urethra and enlargement of the prostate* 2nd Edition. London: Baillière, Tindall and Cox 1902)

with 12 ounces of boracic lotion and the catheter being left in, suprapubic cystotomy was performed. On introducing my finger through the wound, I found the bladder almost filled by a rounded tumour the size of a cricket-ball, which at first I imagined to be an enormous 'middle lobe' of the prostate; but, on closer examination, this was found to be composed of two outgrowths of the lateral lobes projecting into the bladder, each the size of half a cricket ball, with a deep vertical cleft between them, through which the catheter was felt passing into the bladder. A small phosphatic concretion, lying free in the bladder, was removed. The mucous membrane over the most prominent part of the right lobe was then snipped by scissors, the incision enlarged by the finger-nail, and that portion of the lobe easily and rapidly detached from its mucous covering, which was pushed down off it. The prominent portion of the left lobe was similarly dealt with, the whole mass then lying bare of mucous membrane. Each half of this mass was then for convenience broken off by the finger along the line flush with the floor of the bladder, and withdrawn by lithotomy forceps through the suprapubic wound. Their lower portions were found to be quite gangrenous. The main body of the prostate was then attacked and enucleated in its capsule from the sheath and urethra, the finger working its way successively below, outside, above and on the inner side of each lateral lobe, the lobes separating above by the giving way of the superior commisure, and the urethra with its accompanying muscles being peeled off and pushed upwards beneath the pubic arch. The prostate was so large that it blocked the space between the pubic arch and rectum, so that the finger passed round it with some difficulty, strong fibrous bands were met with at the sides and behind the triangular ligament, passing from the sheath to the capsule, which required some force to tear through. The main body of the prostate, now lying loose within its sheath, was tilted to the left beneath the urethra, and delivered into the bladder through the slit made in the mucous membrane in removing the portion of the left lobe projecting into the bladder. A finger of one hand placed in the rectum steadied the prostate during the enucleation and pushed it towards and eventually into the bladder. The prostate was then withdrawn from the bladder by lithotomy foreceps. I would here remark that a very large prostate can be removed whole in this way, owing to the compressibility of the adenomatous tissue of which it is mainly composed. After removal of the prostate the urethra could be traced entire from the triangular ligament to the neck of the bladder surrounding the catheter. Between the fingers in the rectum and that in the cavity whence the prostate had been removed only a thin partition, formed by the wall of the rectum and recto-vesical fascia, could be felt. There was very little bleeding, which was rapidly controlled by irrigation of hot boracic lotion, at the cessation of which the cavity left by removal of the prostate had practically disappeared owing to the rapid contraction of the surrounding tissues. Not a shred of mucous membrane was removed and no sutures were employed in the bladder. No scissors, forceps or cutting instruments of any kind was employed in the enucleation of the prostate, which was entirely effected by the finger. A large drainage-tube was inserted in the bladder and the suprapubic wound sutured by silkworm gut. The usual dressings and large pads of wool for absorption of the urine were applied. The operation lasted half an hour, the patient being three-quarters of an hour under the anaesthetic. The patient stood the operation well, was not in the least collapsed after it and on waking from the anaesthetic commenced to laugh and joke. The temperature never rose above 100°F and remained normal after September 12. The tube was removed in forty-eight hours, after which the bladder was irrigated daily. The sutures were removed on September 12, when the abdominal wound was closed, except where the drainage tube had passed.

On October 7th, 6 ounces of urine were passed naturally by the urethra, after which the quantity discharged in this way gradually increased as the suprapubic wound closed.

On October 16th the patient went for a drive; the fistula had practically closed and he could retain and pass from 12 to 15 ounces of clear, healthy urine naturally.

On November 3rd he returned to France and bore the journey well, but next day there was a leakage of urine by the fistula. This, however, gradually closed and on December 2nd the patient wrote 'I pass my urine quite well by the natural passage and hold my water as long as I like. For instance, last night, from 11.30 pm till 8 this morning (8½ hours) and no urine by the fistula, so really it is a perfect success'.

I pass round for your inspection this enormous prostate, which weighed 10¼ ounces, measuring 5½ inches antero-posteriorly and 3½ inches transversely; also two drawings showing its actual size and physical aspects, as viewed from above and beneath respectively. You will observe that the growth is enveloped by a thin, dense, fibrous capsule which is closely adherent to it. This is the true capsule of the prostate. This is one of the adenomata of which the enlarged prostate is mainly composed and was detached during the removal of the latter. These adenomata, which vary in size from that of a white currant to a greengage, possess separate capsules of their own.'

References

Freyer P J. Clinical lectures on stricture of the urethra and enlargement of the prostate, 2nd Edition. London: Baillière, Tindall and Cox, 1902.
Murphy L P T. The History of Urology. Springfield: Charles C Thomas, 1972.

[40]

Anonymous

Instructive mistakes (1912)

Every surgeon makes mistakes—mistakes in diagnosis, mistakes in judgement, mistakes in operative technique. However, the great majority of us learn from our errors, indeed, this is the true measure of a wise surgeon. We can also learn from the errors of others: 'There, but for the grace of God, go I'. We hear where our colleagues have gone wrong in conversation in the wards, in the changing room and over lunch, at case conferences and at 'death and disaster' meetings, which are now called 'Surgical Audit'. Often one could wish that a larger audience could be exposed to such salutary discussions, but surgeons are more inclined to report their triumphs than disasters, especially in these litigious days. A notable exception was Astley Cooper, who certainly was prepared to publish his surgical errors even when the patient was a peer of the realm (see chapter 22).

A useful, but not often employed, solution is for errors to be published anonymously. When the *British Journal of Surgery* was first published in 1913, it carried a series entitled 'Instructive Mistakes'. This provided a wonderful forum which enabled surgeons, under the cloak of anonymity, to let others learn from their errors. Unfortunately, the onset of the first Great War saw these articles disappear from its pages. Perhaps the time has come for them to reappear.

As fine examples of the value of case reports in instructing us, what better 'Surgical Case Reports from the Past' than these can there be to end this volume?

Anonymous "Instructive mistakes"

British Journal of Surgery 1913; 1: 139–141

'Intussusception mistaken for one of infantile enteritis

William S., aged 10 months. Admitted on August 1, 1912, for diarrhoea and vomiting. On admission the child was rather collapsed and blue; temperature 97°; pulse 130. The child was constantly crying as if in pain. Motions, three or four each day, were greenish, with a little blood and mucus. Vomiting occurred after each feed. A provisional diagnosis of gastro-enteritis was made. Ten drops of brandy and a quarter of a grain of calomel were given every four hours during the first day. From August 2nd to 6th the condition remained much the same as in the last note. The stomach and rectum were washed out twice a day, and a mixture containing bismuth and salol was administered. The stools continued to be loose, and contained both mucus and blood, but were never more frequent than four each day. It was noticed for the first time on August 6, that the abdomen, was distended, and the child was transferred to the surgical side of the hospital. On its arrival there the condition was very grave: pulse 160; respirations 40; temperature 96°; the child being blue and cold. A rather indefinite resistance was felt above the umbilicus. Diagnosis of intussuception was made, and immediate operation resorted to.

Operation (Aug 6, 1912)—Median incision. The common type of ileocolic intusseception was discovered, the apex of the intussuception being in the upper part of the descending colon. A reduction was easily effected and the operation was concluded by performing an appendicostomy through a stab wound. By means of a catheter tied in to this a continuous saline was administered, but the child died twelve hours later.

There can be no doubt that if the nature of this case had been recognized when the child was first admitted it would have had a very good prospect of recovery. Even after five days, and in spite of drugs and purgatives, the invagination of the bowel was readily reducible. The child died as the result of the constant vomiting after food which had continued for six days. The fact that the abdomen showed neither distension nor tumour during the first four days was due to the fact that complete obstruction did not exist. The principal feature which might have prevented this mistake was the scanty nature of the stools. In a case of gastro-enteritis the motions are usually very much more numerous than three or four a day. In this case, although they were only few in number, each stool contained both blood and mucus. Enteritis, on the other hand, rarely causes blood in the stools unless the diarrhoea is very severe.

Internal haemorrhage from a deep epigastric vein in a hernia operation

Frederick P., aged 42, a labourer, was admitted to the hospital for double hernia which had been in existence for about two to three years. He was a thin spare man, with the lax abdominal wall which is associated with certain types of hernia. There was a direct inguinal hernia on both sides, neither of which descended into the scrotum.

Operation (September 9, 1912)—The left side was operated upon first in the ordinary way. The sac had a broad base, and it was pulled well out of the abdomen, clamped with two forceps, and the cut edges sewn together. Otherwise the usual Bassini operation was carried out. The right side was similarly treated, and on separating the structures of the cord from the sac and opening the latter, there was a good deal of free blood. It was naturally thought that this came from one of the spermatic veins, and some time was spent in searching for a wounded vessel. At last it was noticed that the blood was really welling up from the abdomen through the neck of the sac, and at the same time the anaesthetist complained that the patient's pulse was becoming rapid and weak. As it was probable, but not certain, that the intraperitoneal haemorrhage arose from the left operation area, the abdomen was opened by a median incision. The pelvis was full of venous blood, and on mopping this out, the bleeding was found to proceed from one of the deep epigastric veins on the outer extremity of the sutured hernial sac. It was readily secured from within the abdomen, the median incision closed, and the operation completed on the right side. The patient made a good recovery.

This severe internal haemorrhage from one of the deep epigastric veins is an accident the origin of which is easy to understand. The direct hernia had a broad-necked sac, and in pulling this up so as to remove the redundant peritoneum completely, the epigastric vessels must have been lifted up and either cut or torn by the forceps.

It is not so easy to explain why the heamorrhage was into the peritoneum rather than into the tissues of the wound, as the vessel lies outside the peritoneal cavity. The suture which occluded the neck of the sac must have missed its outer part, together with the wounded vein. The conjoined tendon sutured to Poupart's ligament in front of the neck of the sac, prevented the blood from appearing in the wound. It was very fortunate that in this case the necessity of operating on the other side revealed the presence of the internal haemorrhage; otherwise the issue might well have been a fatal one.

Haemorrhage from a ruptured ileocolic artery in the operation for acute appendicitis

Charles W., aged 35, an ironworker. Admitted to hospital with a typical condition of acute appendicitis. He gave a history of three previous attacks, each of about a month's duration, during the past two years. The present attack began three days previously, with abdominal pain and vomiting. A perfectly definite tender mass could be felt low down in the right iliac fossa.

Operation (Nov 4, 1912)—Abdomen opened by a gridiron incision, and an indurated mass exposed formed by the caecum, behind which lay the appendix, pointing almost directly upwards. The appendix was almost entirely gangrenous, and the parts around were infiltrated by inflammatory oedema, but there was no pus. The posterior position of the appendix and the induration of its mesentery made it necessary to pull the caecum downwards and forwards in order to complete the operation. When this had been done in the usual way, bright blood was found to be welling up from depths of the wound. No amount of swabbing through the widely retracted incision revealed the source of the bleeding, and it was necessary therefore to cut through the transverse muscles of the abdomen upwards parallel to the semilunar line.

It was found that the traction on the caecum had torn a large hole in the root of the mesentery, and the ileocolic artery had been ruptured in its terminal part. The bleeding vessel was secured, the hole in the mesentery sewn up, and the wound closed, with drainage. Recovery was uneventful; the drain was removed four days later, and the patient left hospital in four weeks.

The explanation of this accident is readily given. The inflammatory induration, originating in the appendix, had extended to the root of the mesentery, rendering this so friable that it was readily torn by the traction upon the caecum. It is probably wiser in a case of plastic appendicitis to open the abdomen freely by a simple oblique incision, rather than to employ the gridiron opening, which necessitates traction upon the caecum for the exposure of posteriorly situated appendix.'

Reference

Anon. Instructive mistakes. *British Journal of Surgery* 1913: **1**: 139–141.